GREAT BODY FOR KIDS

A Parent's Complete Fitness and Nutritional Guide for Kids

COMMITMENT: the state or quality of being dedicated to a cause, activity, etc. "his commitment to his family"

Chris R. Rea

ReaShape

ISBN: 978-0-9903094-6-8

The nutritional and health information in this book is based on the author's experiences. It is intended only as a guide and is not meant to replace the advice of a physician, dietitian, physical therapist, or other health professional. Always seek competent professional help if you have concerns about the appropriateness of this information for you.

Printed in the United States of America.

For my brother.

Contents

Introduction

For kids today, the times have definitely changed. Our kids have a completely different lifestyle than the kids of yesterday. In the past, children and teenagers had very different types of entertainment and recreation; they leaned much more toward physical activity. Today's entertainment is much less physical. It's much more sedentary—kids watch a lot of TV, play a lot of video games, and spend a lot of time on the computer.

What I am leading to is that today's youth are getting unnecessarily heavy. We now have an overwhelming epidemic of child obesity. About one in three American kids and teens is now overweight or obese, nearly triple the rate in 1963. Childhood obesity is causing kids to have a broad range of health problems that aren't usually seen until adulthood. These include high blood pressure, type 2 diabetes and elevated blood cholesterol levels. It's not just their bodies that are being damaged. Obese children are more prone to low self-esteem, negative body image, and depression.

What's most frightening to me is that being overweight or obese in childhood is linked to earlier death in adulthood. Former Surgeon General Richard Carmona put it very well: "Because of the increasing rates of obesity, unhealthy eating habits and physical inactivity, we may see the first generation that will be less healthy and have a shorter life expectancy than their parents."

As Dr. Carmona pointed out, reduced physical activity is one of the components that has led to such widespread obesity; lack of proper nutrition is another. Eating responsibly and exercising adequately are the necessary steps to take to combat this growing epidemic. In this book, I will cover the physical and psychological steps that parents and guardians can take to help put a stop to childhood obesity. Being overweight has a multitude of negative consequences that, unless properly treated, can last a lifetime.

My adolescent and teenage years were among the best years of my life, primarily because life was so simple and I had so few real responsibilities. The great memories of those years of my life included a lot time that was allocated just to fun. For me, that meant all types of physical activities. I enjoyed playing team and individual sports, but I also enjoyed playing hide and seek, tag, manhunt, and other games with the kids in the neighborhood. Rather than asking my hard-working parents to drive me places, I rode my bike everywhere I could. I rode my bike to school and took myself to the library, to team practice, to visit friends, and to the mall and video arcade.

Kids today often don't walk or ride their bikes to school. They take the bus or their parents drop them off and pick them up. They also get driven everywhere else, including to play dates and sports practice. At home, kids don't play outdoors; they stay inside with their video games. This lack of exercise as a normal, fun part of being a kid or a teen is a big contributor to the vast number of overweight kids. And the fatter a kid gets, the less interested he or she is in being active. This can be the start of lifelong physical and mental problems.

Never could I stress to you enough the importance of engaging in preventive action to avoid these potentially negative consequences. Our youth are our future. We should really take the time to see to it that our kids will be our pride, not our sorrow.

To become successful adults, kids need confidence in themselves. This crucial character trait can easily be lost when kids are embarrassed by their overweight appearance. Sports and physical activity are great ways to build self-confidence, but overweight kids don't participate much in these. When they stay indoors on their computers, they're losing the opportunity to build both a strong, healthy body and the independence and self-confidence that go with it. When parents ask me what they can do to help their kids be stronger and eat better, I don't start with workouts and diets. Instead, I tell them to do whatever they can to improve their child's confidence. That's the number-one priority. Without it, losing weight and getting into shape will be much harder.

1: Nutrition

Proper nutrition is really the backbone of good health for kids. The old saying, "You are what you eat," is as true as it gets. Food is the fuel that generates the energy that makes your body move, breathe, and survive. Just as your car's gasoline has different octanes to measure its potency, your food intake has different potencies as well. High-octane gasoline for your car is the equivalent of high-protein food for your body. Gasoline burns, releasing energy, just as food in your body does. We measure the heat produced when gasoline is burned and the energy that's produced when food is burned in the same unit of heat: a calorie. While your car uses fuel only when the motor is running, your body, even when it's at rest or sleeping, is always consuming calories. Another difference between our bodies and our cars is that once your car's fuel tank is empty, the motor will shut down. Your body is different. If your stomach is empty, your body can't shut down. Instead, it will begin to adjust its metabolism into a more efficient mode and use fuel from its reserve deposits. The reserve deposits in your body are body fat. When the tank in your car is full, you can no longer add any more fuel. However, your body is different. When you eat more food (calories) than you need to fuel your body at the moment, the excess calories get stored as body fat. When your body starts to runs very low on fuel, it taps the stored fat for energy. Storing some energy as fat is very natural and even desirable. The problem comes when you eat so many excess calories that you store a lot of excess fat—and you never stop eating long enough to make your body turn to that excess fat for fuel. That's what makes a kid overweight.

I've been involved in fitness and nutrition for most of my life. As part of my interest and my work, I keep abreast of the latest trends and discoveries concerning nutrition and fitness. I'm always looking for ways to use new information and help people improve their diets and fitness as effortlessly as possible. Year after year, I have kept my body in great shape. Thanks to my constant thirst for knowledge and desire to improve, I have learned ways to make this easier. My motto is "Keep it simple." Being in shape is a lifestyle—it's a marathon, not a sprint. When we choose ways to stay fit, there's no end in sight. Being healthy isn't only about eating right; it's also about exercising and being mentally healthy.

Throughout this book I will talk a lot about exercise, mental health, and an overall healthy lifestyle because I am eager to positively impact our youth. Also, I am an avid promoter of health and fitness for everyone. That includes parents and other adults in a child's life, because I believe it is very important to set a good example. Eating right and exercising truly is my passion. Throughout my career I have been a team coach, a trainer, a nutritionist and a competitive athlete. I have plenty of experience. In this book I'll teach you all about the key components of helping kids getting into shape and stay that way. It really narrows down to nutrition and exercise.

I believe that being a kid is among the best times in our lives. It's a time to have fun, be active, and develop life-long healthy habits. So why not make the most out of this precious period?

Is Your Child at a Healthy Weight?

Combating child obesity starts with proper diet and exercise. But before we get into that, let's talk about your child's weight. Kids normally grow at very different rates. When I was eight, I was actually kind of runty—I was below average for both my height and weight. By the time I was twelve, however, I had started to catch up, and by the time I was fourteen I was above average for my age in height and normal for my weight. Some kids I went to elementary school with were roly-poly when they were in fourth grade and had become much slimmer when they were in seventh grade. Others never really lost that baby weight and stayed overweight all through high school and beyond.

I've noticed that when the parents are overweight themselves, they're less likely to see their child as overweight, even when he or she clearly is much heavier than other kids their age and height. It's hard to be objective about your own child. If you think your kid is overweight, it's hard to know where he or she is on the normal weight range for height and age.

Is it time to worry or not? One good way to find out is to check the body mass index percentile calculator for kids and teens created by the federal Centers for Disease Control. You can use the calculator by going to the CDC website at apps.nccd.cdc.gov/dnpabmi/.

The calculator will ask for your child's age, sex, weight, and height. After you enter these values, it will calculate your child's body mass index and then find the corresponding BMI-for-age percentile for the child's age and sex. The BMI-for-age percentile shows how your child's weight compares to that of other children of the same age and sex. So, if your child's BMI-for-age percentile is 65 percent, that means that she's heavier than 65 percent of other girls of the same age.

The percentiles work out like this:

Underweight: less than the 5th percentile

Healthy weight: 5th percentile up to the 85th percentile

Overweight: 85th percentile to less than the 95th percentile

Obese: 95th percentile or greater

Generally speaking, if you kid falls into the healthy weight range, your focus should be on staying there with a healthy diet. If your child is above or below the healthy weight range, that doesn't mean he or she needs to go on an official diet. Instead, your focus should be on moving the kid's diet—and your family's—in a healthier direction.

Feed Your Kids Right

As a child I simply ate whatever was fed to me; I pretty much liked it all. Fortunately, my mother was a great cook! My parents come from

Spain, where people take tremendous pride in their wonderful and varied cuisine. Whenever we went to Spain to visit our extended family, I always ate everything at the excellent meals we had. These extravagant meals were always delicious and made with the highest-quality ingredients. They were sometimes higher in calories, especially from sweets, than was necessarily best for me, but we only had meals like that on special occasions. My health and activity levels as a child were definitely great, thanks to good food and an ample amount of exercise. Up until my freshman year in high school, I was oblivious to anything about my own nutrition.

Many kids today aren't as fortunate as I was. Among other things, they don't eat much home cooking. They have busy moms who find that eating out at fast food restaurants, ordering out for pizza, or serving microwave meals is quicker and easier than cooking. Kids today also have a lot less time for just playing outside, riding their bikes, and other activities. Seeing so many kids today who are out of shape has given me the drive to help this nationwide problem.

Overweight and obese kids suffer so much and so unnecessarily. The psychological effects of child obesity are very damaging. Fat kids are teased and even bullied. They feel self-conscious about their bodies, which can lead them to hide indoors with their video games and be even less physically active. Even at a young age, their quality of life isn't high. I cannot stress enough the importance of quality of life, which begins with the most important aspect: good health. Health is something many of us take for granted. Most of us assume that, because we live here in the U.S., we must already have good health. This is definitely not the case at all—actually, quite the contrary. Most people in this country exercise less than people in most other countries, even though we know that even simple exercises such as walking are very good for our health. We'd rather drive than walk even a few blocks.

Exercise, proper nutrition, and a positive attitude are all healthy habits that any kid can learn. Whenever I hear someone say, "I can't do that, I can't diet, I can't exercise," what he is really saying is that he is either too lazy to make the sacrifices or that he lacks the confidence to believe that his goals can be accomplished. All too often, we are our own worst enemy; our minds are full of tricks and deception. We begin to believe outlandish thoughts and ideas, outright lies and deception. Don't feel singled out, because we all fall victim to this. Even the best of us fall into this category! This is why even the best athletes have coaches and experts to assist them to reach their goals and perform at the highest level at all times. Having a coach or mentor who motivates you or teaches you how to reach your best performance is an effective way to assist you in reaching your goals. As we go further into this book, I will continue to mention the importance of having proper guidance while working to achieve your fitness goals.

Child obesity is a broad dilemma. The problem goes far and beyond simple changes in nutrition and exercise. To effectively tackle this problem, we must get to its core.

The roots of childhood weight problems often begin very early on, way before a child is obviously too heavy. Although the problem actually begins at a very young age, we must never waste time blaming anyone or anything. Making excuses or justifying yourself is not an effective means of helping your child.

Let's not worry too much about what caused the problem. Rather, let's use our energies to find treatments and solutions to it as well as preventive measures to avoid us from repeating the same mistakes. Never should anyone dwell on mistakes and reasons for past failures, problems. and shortcomings. This is such a tremendous waste of precious time, energy, and resources. Instead, harness all your energy to conquer or treat these problems.

Overweight kids today face the true core of this problem: lack of confidence in themselves. Confidence is such a valuable attribute to have. Plainly put, confidence is everything. It is the key ingredient on the recipe for success. Believing in yourself is what it takes to bring yourself to the next level. As a competitive athlete for most of my life, I was taught confidence early on by every coach I had. Unfortunately, it didn't really sink in for me until later on in my life, at the tail end of my competitive athletic career.

Now, please understand that by no means am I a psychologist. This book is about combating child obesity through diet and exercise. It may seem that when I talk about confidence I'm straying from the topic of child obesity, but not at all. Kids being overweight is a tremendous problem. Just like any other problem, we must attack it from the core to effectively conquer it. Overweight kids suffer tremendously, including psychologically.

For this book to work effectively for you and your family, let's start from the very beginning. Let's assume if you have purchased this book, you are most likely the parent to one or more overweight kids.

Overweight youths are missing out on so much that it is truly a shame. As a parent, you can help change this. The good thing about being overweight is that it is reversible, unlike a childhood disease such as diabetes. A child who is obese must be taught there is light at the end of the tunnel. The child must learn that there is an effective process that will return him or her to being what they always wanted to be, and that is to be just a regular child. Being a kid that is overweight is no easy task. These kids are subject to mental abuse that comes in from many directions. You as a parent might reprimand your child if he or she eats too much; their friends and peers tease or ignore them for being heavy. Nobody picks the heavy kids to be part of their team or star in the school play. This is sad. Most people and many parents out there don't even realize all how much residual psychological damage occurs throughout these childhood years. Kids are extremely fragile. Much care needs to be taken during these crucial formative years.

The way adults behave is largely due to their childhood and up-bringing. Think of a tree once it is planted. This tree needs proper care and nourishment in order for it to grow strong. The same applies to kids. They need a lot of attention in so many different ways to develop in a healthy manner.

I am sure you're now thinking, what does this have to do with childhood obesity? By the end of this book, this will not only all makes sense, but it will be simple for you to implement the diet, workouts, and mental coaching techniques and strategies to further help you, your children, or anyone else. My effective techniques for getting into great physical shape are proven methods to success. Throughout the years I have kept myself in great shape while being mentally sharp as well. I am a strong believer in being well-rounded because this will not only improve your quality of life, but also make you a more productive. Proper nutrition and training leads to a sharper mind and more confidence. With more confidence, so many more doors will be open for you.

I will be teaching you and your children how to properly eat and exercise not just to be in fantastic shape but also to do well in school, sports, and social activities. Your child's social skills will most definitely improve as a result of what you're about to learn. Yes, of course, I will teach you about weight loss and being in shape, but what the big picture really requires is the magical word confidence. That's what we will learn, develop, and cultivate. Once confidence is developed, all of your children's goals are within reach. There are plenty of diet books on the market; many of them are excellent, many are not. However, the way my approach differs is that I stress confidence and ways to acquire it. Increased confidence is needed to win because, without it, the victories will not happen at all. It starts within the mind.

The Psychology Behind It All

Of course, it begs the question: how important is it for us to be so preoccupied with our children's optimum physical health? Parents often think, "Why not let kids be kids" when it comes to snacks such as sweets or any other treats. Parents often believe that kids should have fun. They figure that eating any sort of treat they want between meals is fine, as long as the children eat the main course at meals. I strongly agree that kids shouldn't be pressured into eating as if they were on an extremely restricted diet. Growing, active kids are hungry and need some between-meal snacks.

During my collegiate years as a competitive wrestler, I had to drop a substantial amount of weight through a 16-week low-carbohydrate diet. I don't recommend that to anyone but a highly competitive athlete, but even now I maintain a low-carb diet that I find quite easy to follow. The average person may find it too radical. For dieting and training, the choices are entirely up to the individual. My rule of thumb is simple. Choose a meal and exercise program your child can follow for the long run. The goal should be to make it possible for your children to reach their fitness goals. For example, if your goal is for your child to stay in decent shape, then a moderate meal and exercise program is suggested. If you want your child to compete at high levels in a sport, then another meal and exercise program would need to be followed. For most parents and kids, everyday goals may be better and more realistic. Everyday goals could include being able to wear off-the-rack clothing (not from the husky department), or just not gaining any more weight, or feeling energetic enough to go for a bicycle ride. These choices and goals would be entirely up to you and your child—the goals are the things that are important to you. I've found that for most overweight kids, the most common goal is to be fit enough and slim enough so that they don't stand out—they want to just blend in with the other kids. Amazing, isn't it, that a goal could be so simple. yet there are so many overweight kids today? To simply blend in and be like everyone else is really not that difficult, but unfortunately we make it much more complicated than we have to.

As parents we really need to step up and take responsibility for our children's weight problems, health issues, and decreased self-esteem. Parents need accept responsibility for their children's problems because, at the very beginning, kids are really innocent victims. When kids are small, they often crave the foods that their mothers ate during pregnancy. For example, if, during pregnancy, the mother consumed a lot of sweets, then later on the child craves the same foods. Another example of mothers behaving responsibly during their pregnancy smoking.

Kids whose mothers smoked during pregnancy have a higher chance of suffering from certain mental illnesses, such as bipolar depression and attention deficit disorder. Kids who grow up breathing secondhand smoke are more likely to get asthma and frequent respiratory illnesses. Kids whose mothers drank heavily during pregnancy can have lifelong learning and emotional disabilities. Yes, there is treatment and medication for these disorders, but the real problem is that most go on for years without being diagnosed or treated. In other words, a lifetime can go by and the child may never realize that his or her quality of life was both hindered and suppressed. They never got the chance to live out the life they could have had. To tackle the growing epidemic of child obesity, we must tackle these problems right from their inception. Kids need a healthy environment right from the start.

Starting Off the Right Way

While the unborn child is in the womb, it gets nourishment from the food that the mother eats. The pregnant mother's diet can vary drastically with the quality of food that is consumed. The old term, "she's eating for two," doesn't mean that the woman must consume large amounts of food during her pregnancy in order for her child to be properly nourished. Rather, the pregnant and soon-to-be mother should closely monitor what she is eating, because her child's health depends largely on her food intake. A pregnant mother should closely monitor her food intake, right down to the calories and protein, complex and simple carbohydrates, and fats (saturated, trans, polyunsaturated, monounsaturated and omega-3). She should be consuming proper amounts of high-quality food. The proper amount of calories, grams of fat, and carbohydrates should be taken into consideration while preparing a meal plan, in order to ensure the child's best possible health. Eating foods that are not balanced, or that are too high in saturated fat or trans fat, will also hinder the child's health later in life.

It is also a very wise decision for pregnant women to remain active during pregnancy. Walking, shopping, and basic house chores are considered light forms of exercise which have been proven to be very beneficial for not only a healthy pregnancy but a healthier and more active baby as well. Many pregnant women follow exercise programs designed to help them stay fit and build muscle tone without endangering the baby. Doctors recommend pregnancy exercise, but they stress it needs to be safe, regular, moderate exercise. Strenuous workouts, even if you did them before pregnancy, aren't good for you now. The safest activities during pregnancy are swimming and walking. You're not likely to hurt yourself doing these activities. If you feel comfortable doing them, you can keep them up until close to your delivery date. After delivery, regular exercise helps you lose any excess weight you're still carrying from the pregnancy. It keeps you in the habit of staying fit and sets a great example for your kids as they grow up.

Speeding Up Your Metabolism

Speeding up your body's metabolism—the way it uses energy—is a process that simply doesn't happen overnight; it can take months of constant exercise. The benefit of increasing your body's metabolism is that your body runs more efficiently. An increased metabolism has two major benefits: you can ingest more calories without gaining body fat, and you become more active by having more energy throughout the day. These two benefits alone should convince you to take the necessary steps in order to increase your body's metabolism. Your body's genetics also plays a role in the speed of your metabolism. Some people just naturally run at higher or lower metabolic speeds.

The goal is never to eat until you feel really full or stuffed. The desire to overeat is very strong. For most of human history, getting barely enough to eat was the norm. Because we didn't know where or when our next meal was coming, we instinctively eat as much as possible when food is plentiful. That worked out well for people at a time when food was always scarce, but in our modern world, food is everywhere. Our bodies still can't quite believe it, however, and push us to eat more whenever we can. To counteract this natural tendency to overeat, we need to make a conscious effort and be very aware of what sorts of foods we're choosing and how and when we eat them.

Proper meal planning is a necessary factor for increasing your body's metabolism. The frequency of your meals is important, as is the size of your portions. The types of foods you eat are equally important. You want to make sure you get a good balance of proteins, carbohydrates (sugary and starchy foods), and good dietary fats.

Food Components

Protein	Carbohydrates	Fiber	Fat
lean meats	potato	vegetables	nuts
fish	rice	fruit	vegetable oils
egg whites	pasta	beans	avocado
protein powder	oatmeal		

Eating a balanced meal means choosing a food from each category at every meal. I will give you an example of a complete day of healthy eating in the chart below. I suggest spacing your meals roughly two to four hours apart. Eating right is partly a matter of trial and error. In time, you will figure out what food choices work best for you.

Drinking is just as important as eating. An adult should aim to drink two to three quarts of plain water daily. Coffee, tea, herbal tea, soda, and other beverages are fine as long as they're unsweetened or sweetened with artificial sweeteners. Avoid fruit juice with added sugar in the form of high-fructose corn syrup. If you want to drink juice, select 100 percent fruit juice and thin it by at least half with plain water.

There are so many food choices and combinations you can choose from. When you begin to eat in this balanced manner, you will immediately feel positive changes: increased energy, improved sleep, and improved complexion.

Whenever possible, get your fruits and vegetables from local farmer's markets. Try to purchase wild-caught fish instead of farm-raised fish. Try to buy as much organically grown food as possible, especially the meats and eggs. Who knows what the future will bring upon our health if we constantly eat foods that are doused with chemicals and preservatives? Being a pregnant mom is enough of a responsibility. Why not make the best of it by eating right and exercising moderately in order to make the experience as easy as possible? At the same time, you'll be providing your child with the best possible start in life.

Successful people lead by example; this is a time-proven method. As a college wrestling coach, I wanted my athletes to perform at the highest levels so they would win. For me motivate the team members to reach that level, I had to be able to do everything I asked them to do, even the most difficult exercise routines. If I just sat back with a whistle in my mouth and a protruding stomach, I am sure the team would have respected me less and not given their very best efforts. Never could I stress enough the importance of teamwork and leading by example. Remember that your family is your team and you are one of their coaches.

After the baby is born, an entirely new format of nutrition and exercise for both the mother and child needs to be implemented. Research has shown that children born from a lean mother are much more active than children born from overweight mothers. A healthy baby is one with a good appetite, but having a good appetite is only a part of being healthy. The old philosophy of forcing your child to eat has been proven to be ineffective for raising a healthy child. Breastfeeding as much as possible in the baby's first year is usually the best approach. Breastfed babies seem to be less likely to become obese later on in life. Breastfeeding has two great advantages over formula. The first is nutrition. Mother's milk provides the perfect combination of fat, carbohydrates, and protein for the baby's needs. It is always a good rule of thumb to presume that anything natural is better than synthetic.

Portion Control

Portion control is a tremendously overlooked factor in meal planning. The quality of the food is just as important as the quantity that is consumed. People are often under the impression that as long as they are eating healthy foods, they won't gain weight. This is not true at all. We either gain or lose weight depending on the calories we burn. Oatmeal is a healthy food, but eat three bowls a day and eventually you will gain weight! Peanut butter is another great example, because it is very nutritious but is extremely high in calories. Therefore, anything more than one or two spoonfuls and you might be ingesting too many calories.

Babies instinctively control their own portions, eating enough to feel satisfied and then stopping. Infants only overeat if their caretakers force food on them. Breastfed babies tend to be less likely to become overweight or binge eaters later in life, perhaps because they learned to control their portions from birth. Children who overeat or binge tend to have developed that trait during their younger years. Often it's because their caretakers pressured them to eat or used food as a reward to entice them into eating more. Techniques such as rewarding children to eat more vegetables by promising them sweets, or penalizing them by not allowing dessert if they don't finish their main course or their vegetables don't really work. In fact, they can backfire, leading kids to associate food with reward or punishment. This leads to obesity and lowered self-esteem and may even contribute to eating disorders such as anorexia or bulimia.

Proper childhood nutrition begins right at home. A child who develops proper eating habits early on is much more likely to continue this healthy pattern as the years pass. Once good nutrition is embedded into the child's psyche, it is been proven to greatly reduce their chances of becoming obese.

2: It All Begins at Home

As the child grows, it will be influenced in many ways, including nutritionally, by the example the parents set. Children are quite impressionable. At this important time in their lives, parents must take advantage of that in a positive way by impressing good habits, such as diet and exercise. While at home the entire family should try to always eat together—beginning and finishing the meal at the same time. This is also a great time to bond. Never should there be any distractions while eating, such as a television, radio, computer, or telephone. Family meals should be dedicated to the family alone.

The time in the child's life right before school begins (usually between the ages of two and five) is especially effective for the family to eat the same healthy foods together. This teaches the child at an early age which foods are nutritious. Food portions should entirely be up to each individual. The meals should be prepared "family style," meaning that the various dishes should be placed in the middle of the table with serving spoons or passed around. Each person, including the children, helps him or herself to whatever amount of each dish is desired. Instead of giving the child a fixed portion of each food by filling the plate for him, serving family style lets the child choose the amount that satisfies him. When the plate is filled for the child, the child feels pressured to eat everything on it—and maybe even be directly told by a parent to eat it all. This keeps the child from learning how to sense that he's full and want to stop eating. In the long run, this can lead to overeating and obesity. It can also lead to arguing at the table about food, which can later lead to unhealthy eating and behavior patterns.

In family style serving, everyone at the table chooses the portion that best suits his or her appetite and personal preferences. Parents sometimes worry that a child won't eat portions large enough, or won't enough variety, for this approach to provide good nutrition. In fact, children will never under nourish themselves. From birth, they have a instinctive ability to know how much they should eat. They may not seem to eat enough at each meal, but often that is a parent applying an adult's perspective to portion size. If you kid is hungry, he or she will instinctively eat enough to satisfy that hunger—and no more. Likewise, a child might not eat all her vegetables at one meal, but will make up for it another.

Parents often can't seem to understand this and make the grave mistake of trying to force-feed their children. This method not only doesn't work, but it backfires as well by making the child begin to think that eating is a chore and without any enjoyment. Other negative consequences can also occur. The child learns how to manipulate and bargain with the parents for different foods, desserts, or privileges.

Another improper technique parents perform is to reward their children for eating. A mother might say, for example, "Mmmm, these vegetables are tasty," or "Wow! I am so proud of you for eating your vegetables." Or she might say, "Eat your vegetables and you can have a cookie" or "You cleaned your room! Have some have potato chips." These unsuccessful methods only lead to negative consequences, such as increased obesity and lower self-esteem, later on.

Balanced Meals

Meals should always be balanced, meaning that they provide a good ratio of fats, carbohydrates, and protein. They should also be balanced in terms of frequency and regularity. Family meals should consist of the basic three meals—breakfast, lunch, and dinner. In addition, up to three healthy snacks a day are fine—growing kids get hungry, and some kids are more hungry than others.

Breakfast is the day's first meal. It should consist of foods that will quickly enter your system and provide immediate energy to your body.

This energy is needed because you body has gone without eating the entire time you were asleep. After hours without food, you wake up hungry and craving foods that will provide quick energy. You might want something sweet, like breakfast cereal, the most popular breakfast in America. The problem with cereal and other popular breakfast foods, such as toaster pastries or pancakes, is that they are refined carbohydrates. They get digested quickly and enter your bloodstream as glucose (blood sugar). That does give you some quick energy, but it can also give you a quick energy crash a couple of hours later. Your blood sugar drops and you feel tired and also hungry. But do you want your kid to get an energy crash during math class in the morning? Of course not. To avoid the crash, your kid needs a better breakfast that's more balanced. Instead of breakfast cereal, aim for a breakfast that has complex carbohydrates, protein, and fat. Scrambled eggs with buttered whole-wheat toast, for instance, gives your child a better start to the day. So does a bowl of old-fashioned oatmeal (not the instant kind) with raisins and a bit of milk. Her blood sugar will go up more smoothly after eating a nutritious meal that doesn't get absorbed too quickly, and it will stay on a more even keel for several hours.

It's also important to take in fluids at breakfast and with every meal. Kids shouldn't be taking in caffeine in large amounts, so coffee and tea are out. Water is the best and least expensive choice. Milk is OK if your child can digest it—many kids lose their ability to digest milk by the time they are eight.

For breakfast, people always ask me how much juice is OK. My answer is always the same: not very much. Fruit juice is simply concentrated sugar—often with added high-fructose corn syrup to make it even sweeter. Eat fresh fruit instead when possible.

Remember that sugar is only an emergency form of energy and should only be consumed when the body really needs it, such as after a workout or at breakfast if you feel very hungry. Have you ever noticed what happens to sugar when it is cooked or heated, such as when a cake is baked? The sugar caramelizes and turns brown. That's great for a cake, but when it happens inside your body, that's not so great. The sugar sticks to your cells and clogs up the tiny blood vessels that bring oxygen and nutrients to your organs, such as your kidneys and eyes. Think of eating candy and how that gives you cavities in your teeth. Well, the same applies to your body when sugar is consumed.

You might think that artificial sweeteners are good alternative to natural sugar. In small amounts every now and then, artificial sweeteners are fine. I recommend against using them frequently. Artificial sweeteners tend to make you retain fluid and bloat up. Also, research has shown that people who drink artificially sweetened soda actually gain more weight than people who drink sugary soda. The reason is that the artificial sweetener provides sweetness without calories. That's the point, right? Yet when you drink something sweet and don't get any nutrition from it, that triggers your body to want more calories. In particular, it triggers sugar cravings.

Think of a recovering alcoholic. An alcoholic needs to refrain from drinking alcohol because he cannot control his consumption. In order for his/her recovery to be successful, that person can no longer drink any alcohol. Why? Because with just one drink the alcoholic's brain will sense that special taste and, remembering that it was enjoyed in the past, demand much more. The same is true with sugar. If you go a long time without eating sweet foods, you begin to forget about your craving for them. But if you use an artificial sweetener, your body remembers how much it likes sugar and begins to crave it again. The best tactic is avoid or sharply limit your use of artificial sweeteners.

If you really miss the sweet taste of sugar in your coffee or in other ways, and feel you much use an artificial sweetener, I recommend stevia, an all-natural zero-calorie sugar substitute made from the leaves of a South American plant.

To reduce your craving for sweets, it is best to eat low-glycemic carbohydrates regularly throughout the day. These are carbohydrates that are absorbed slowly, such as whole grains, fruit, and beans. This keeps your blood sugar at a steady level, instead of spiking up and suddenly dropping. Sugar also temporarily "revs up" a child. Avoid giving your children sugary or high-glycemic foods at night. They can keep them from falling asleep.

When your child is a toddler is a great time to set the proper foundation for nutrition by not giving him or her sugary foods. They won't miss sugar later on if they don't get much of it now. We all need some type of sweets in our system both for energy and as a treat. Fresh fruit the absolute best option for dessert and for snacks. Milk also provides sugar in the form of lactose, or milk sugar. Once your child becomes used to milk, fresh fruit, and other natural foods for sweetness, then he or she has less of a propensity to crave concentrated sweets such as candy and cookies.

Water

Newborn babies are designed to drink breast milk or formula if necessary. Aside from breast milk or the equivalent, which we usually stop having before age three, we are designed to drink water—and only water. Not fruit juice, not soda, and not energy drinks.

Two to four quarts (8 to 16 cups) per day seems to be the perfect quantity, depending upon your activity level and body size. Most people can actually drink less than that if they also eat lots of foods that naturally contain water, such as fruits and vegetables. Water does wonders for your body by replenishing your cells, improving your skin, flushing the body's organs, and, of course, quenching thirst. I suggest that you only serve water or possibly unsweetened herbal tea at family meals.

Meal Planning for the Family

Protein	Carbohydrates	Fiber	Fats
chicken breast	sweet potato	fruits	avocado
turkey breast	brown rice	vegetables	coconut
egg whites	oatmeal	whole-grain pasta	olive oil

whey protein powder	oat bran	beans	canola oil
fish (wild caught)	high-fiber bran cereal		peanuts
lean red meat			almonds
low-fat milk			cashews
low-fat cottage cheese			walnuts

For the average adult, choosing one food from each of the food groups listed above for each meal. Of course, you can choose other options aside from the ones I list here. Here are some examples:

Daily Menu for Adults

Breakfast	2 egg whites, 1 yolk, scrambled
	fruit
	2/3 cup old-fashioned oatmeal
Snack	1 protein bar
Lunch	grilled chicken breast
	steamed vegetables
	sweet potato
Snack	almonds
	fruit
Dinner	broiled salmon
	whole-grain pasta
	broccoli
	green salad with olive oil and vinegar
Snack	low-fat Greek yogurt with blueberries

Vary your choices and find the options that satisfy you. Learning how to eat will render huge dividends in terms of maintaining great health with your family. The next examples are daily meal plans for a vegan adult (a vegan is someone who doesn't eat any animal foods) and for a vegetarian who doesn't eat meat.

Daily Menu for Adult Vegan

Breakfast	1 scoop of soy protein isolate mixed with oatmeal and a banana
Snack	walnuts fruit
Lunch	noodles with peanut sauce green salad with almonds
Snack	carrot and celery sticks
Dinner	steamed tofu steamed mixed vegetables sweet potato
Snack	peanut butter blended with 1 scoop soy protein isolate

Daily Menu for Adult Vegetarian

Breakfast	3/4 cup egg whites, scrambled high-fiber bran cereal
Snack	1 cup low-fat cottage cheese
Lunch	light tuna with green salad
Snack	1 cup low-fat Greek yogurt
Dinner	steamed fish broccoli rabe steamed with garlic
Snack	1/2 cup raisins

Remember that there is always an option that is healthy for everyone. You will quickly learn how to make the best choices for family meals that are as healthy and tasty as possible. (Later in this book you will see, in greater detail, the many different meal options.) I have taken into consideration the fact that most children don't like eating vegetables. I've found ways to alter and improve their taste, making them palatable for the kids to eat. Never is it a wise idea to feed your family "prepared" meals. They may be convenient and taste great, but these packaged meals are loaded with added sodium (salt) and a lot of hidden sugar.

Even if they claim to be low-fat or low-calorie, this does not mean they're healthy. The best quality meals are the ones that are prepared at home, because you can control which foods go into the recipe of your choice.

The mistake many people make is to prepare or buy food only according to taste. Food should be bought primarily for its nutritional value. Cost is also a factor. But inexpensive, highly nutritious foods also taste great! Choose your food for its nutritional value first, then cost, and finally the taste. The chart below is an example of a full day of healthy eating for an adult.

Healthy Eating for an Adult

Example 1

Breakfast	1 cup Fiber One cereal with strawberries and low-fat milk
Snack	1 peanut butter high-fiber protein bar
Lunch	light tuna with low-calorie mayonnaise on a whole-wheat, high-fiber English muffin
Snack	1 fruit
Dinner	chicken breast parmigiana made with all-natural tomato sauce broccoli sautéed with olive oil and garlic sugar- and fat-free frozen yogurt
Snack	almonds

Example 2

Breakfast	high-fiber waffles with sugar-free syrup
Snack	whey protein isolate shake with peanut butter
Lunch	chicken breast on whole-grain bread with nonfat cheese and lettuce
Snack	fruit
Dinner	whole-grain lasagna green salad with olive oil and vinegar dressing
Snack	low-fat Greek yogurt

Your children will most likely be picky eaters—most kids are, at least about some foods. Do not fall into their manipulation traps by giving them only the food they want! Kids will eat anything and they will never starve with the foods you give them. They may not like one meal you prepared, but they will most likely enjoy the next. The key is to always cook healthy foods because, by doing this, you will accomplish so much more than just to keep them fit; you will raise their confidence, which is the ultimate goal!

Identifying your child's overall needs is extremely important, especially when they are not yet able to speak to you. Babies have different cry tones and each tone calls for something different. The parent must learn to identify which cry tones indicate that the baby is asking for food, affection, and diaper changes (just to name a few). When your child wants attention, it's not the same as wanting food, but parents can easily confuse the two and end up giving a child food when what she needs is cuddling. Children raised in orphanages have a higher malnutrition and death rate than those raised with parents. What this means is that giving your child sufficient attention and affection will enable him to grow healthier, both physically and mentally, while enabling you to communicate more efficiently with him. Communication is the basis for every successful relationship. Communication with your child goes far and beyond simple day-to-day parlays. Successful communication includes respecting her decisions when eating, and allowing her to eat the amount she wants. Most of the time, the child will eat the necessary amount of food. But some children may eat too much or sneak in unhealthy snacks throughout the day. If the children are fed responsibly, chances are that they are less likely to desire unhealthy snacks. Whenever we crave sweets, it is because we don't have sufficient sugar in our bloodstream. This comes not from too little sugar but from too little complex carbohydrates throughout the day. In order to avoid craving sweets, we must eat a sufficient amount of complex carbohydrates, such as whole grain breads and brown rice. Are you noticing that all roads lead to cooking responsibly with high-quality, balanced meals? Preparing nutritional meals will simply improve your family's day. That type of cooking will provide adequate nutrition with a high energy level. Your family will avoid the tiredness and bad moods that come from blood sugar crashes caused by eating too many highly refined carbohydrates.

In early childhood, setting the right example of good nutrition is crucial. A mistake now may set the pace for years ahead. At this age, a child will be very accepting of the foods he is fed. That's why it is so important for you parents to really get involved and educate yourselves about proper nutrition. Most parents really have no idea about eating for maximum performance. Parents innocently cook and prepare their family's meals primarily based on taste and convenience, automatically assuming that the meal is healthy. This is an extremely common mistake, because most people simply don't have the nutritional knowledge to make better choices for themselves and their families. Look at a simple dinner such as baked chicken with potatoes and sautéed spinach. Is that healthy meal? Yes and no. If you drown the baked potato in sour cream and butter, you're adding a lot of calories to it; if you don't eat the skin, you're losing out on the fiber and extra minerals. If you top the spinach with cheese, you're also adding extra calories. If you serve a rotisserie chicken from the store, you're giving your kids a lot of extra salt from the barbecue sauce—and a lot of extra sugar if they drench the chicken with ketchup. If thinking that it is a healthy meal. Simplest is best. Remember that food is fuel! And you are what you eat!

3: Preschoolers

The preschooler is out to learn and grow in all areas of his life. Eating is definitely no exception. Unlike a newborn or toddler, the preschooler is purposeful. The preschooler has a sense of what he or she can or can't do, and is eager and willing to try new challenges and adventures. These kids have a feeling of what they can accomplish and what is permissible. However, they are still children and you will need to accommodate to their unique childness.

Preschoolers are trying to learn and to impress their parents. They begin to be able to hold their own fork and knife and even hold a glass without dropping it because their muscles are becoming stronger. Preschoolers develop at a very fast rate, but their coordination lags behind the rest of their growth. Involving your kid in age-appropriate coordination-improving activities helps him develop coordination naturally and in a fun way.

Any activities to develop coordination, however, build skills only for that particular activity. The more activities you try, the better coordination and conditioning will become, and the more fun you and your kid will have. It's all about variety. Another factor that should be considered when kids engage in a multitude of activities is that the old saying stands true: "The jack of all trades is the master of none." This means that if the preschooler is involved in everything, it is unlikely that he or she will become really good at any one activity, talent, or sport. Is that important at age four? Not really. I truly believe that it is quite all right for a preschooler to be involved in a lot of different things. The child may not ace any particular activity or show much talent for it, but he's learning where his natural aptitudes and interests lie. He's also learning to feel a sense of accomplishment and success. This is a great way for a child to discover his true interests and passions. This is the trial-and-error method and it works quite effectively. Another advantage for the kids is the social aspect of activities such as gymnastics and just going to the playground. The more activities that they are involved with, the more people and friends they will meet. The more people that you and your children meet, the more positive socialization will happen. Your kid will learn to interact well with other kids and adults. I am also a strong advocate of a household filled with soccer balls, basketballs, bikes, and dancing. A happy and athletically friendly household has an energetic vibe.

Preschoolers are growing fast. Now's the time to put them on the right path for healthy eating. Preschoolers need a higher fat diet than that of teenagers and adults. As the children age, their requirements of dietary fat decrease.

Meal Plan for a Preschooler

Breakfast	oatmeal
	high-fiber English muffin
Snack	handful of raisins
Lunch	grilled cheese sandwich
	high-fiber English muffin
Snack	banana
Dinner	hamburger made with lean ground beef on
	high-fiber bun broccoli with melted cheese
Snack	hard-boiled omega-3 egg with high-fiber bread

Exercise for Preschoolers

Exercise is just as important as eating properly and resting sufficiently. Today's kids are much less active than in the past. Computers have a lot to do with this problem because these kids can literally spend hours in front of the computer or TV playing games or Web surfing. Parents need to keep this to a minimum and encourage activity instead.

Exercise is extremely important for a multitude of reasons, ranging from being physically fit to increasing overall confidence. Kids' exercise programs are very simple to construct because free time, healthy energetic friends, and plenty of school activities are always available to them. Once again, parents need to get involved in order to see to it that the kids are involved in the physical activities that the kids enjoy most. It is very important for them to have fun, no matter what sport or activity they are involved in.

Let's think about having fun for a minute. As adults, we want careers that we enjoy. We choose a spouse because we enjoy being with him or her. We pursue hobbies and activities that we enjoy. Right? The truth is that we will never be very successful at something if we don't have a passion for it.

Parents often overlook what their children's gifts and interests are, and lead them into sports that they enjoy themselves. In actuality, the parents should closely watch the children as they play, gathering information, to see what the child's natural gifts and interests are. All kids need exercise, regardless of whether they're really interested in it or not. Yes, some kids will have no interest in sports or even being outdoors. They seem to be lazy or unmotivated, but there's more to it than that; don't blame the child. These children are a challenge for parents, but there is hope and light at the end of the tunnel. First, ask yourself if you are setting a good example of being active yourself and planning fun family activities. If you are also a couch potato, no amount of telling your child to go out and ride his bike will get his attention. If you're active and your child isn't, you need to really pay close attention, without giving the impression to the child that you are being controlling. Every kid has something physical he or she likes to do; you just need to figure out what it is and present it as a choice, not something you are forcing on the child. If the child senses that you are trying to control him, he will become withdrawn, making it even more difficult for you to reach him and for him to trust you. A breach of respect is something that we never want.

Children are delicate mechanisms. When a child seems withdrawn, unmotivated, or lazy, parents must continue to set a good example and never give up. We all have a gift, something that we are good at. We have a limited lifetime to figure out what it is. Helping a child discover what her gift or passion is can begin early in life with the careful help of the parents. Parents can carefully and patiently observe the kid's behavior. Eventually the child's passions, interests, and gifts will become clear. Even with activities your kid enjoys, the secret is to always make them seem like fun, rather than mandatory. It is all about the presentation and communication with your child.

Workouts for Muscle Strength

Cardio Exercises
Any sport that involves running, such as soccer, football, tennis

Strength and Muscle-Building Exercises
For kids over age 8, these exercises can be done every other day; make sure there is always a rest day in between.

5 sets push-ups   8 to 10 repetitions
5 sets free squats or lunges   10 repetitions
25 sit-ups

When children perform these exercises, it is important to carefully monitor them to see that they are doing them safely. There has always been a myth that if children perform strength and muscle-building exercises, they can stunt their growth or weaken their bones. This has been proven to be untrue. In fact, just the opposite: All types of exercise has been proven to help kids develop both physically and mentally.

Once again, I must stress to you the power of leading by example. Parents should be involved. Not only will this benefit everyone physically but it will also enhance the emotional bond. You will be spending more quality time together and you will have more things in common to share, discuss, and experience. Bonding among fellow athletes is also important. When you all endure the same struggles, you experience defeats and victories in a way that only a competitive athlete can understand. These are all positive, confidence-building experiences. Parents have no idea really how much they truly influence the well-being of their children and how much their kids really look up to them. That's why it's so important for parents to get involved with their kids' activities. This benefits the parents as well, because they need to be in shape; they also need to maintain a youthful spirit. Parents should not look at this as a burden, but rather, an opportunity to have fun, get into shape, and develop a positive drive.

4: The School-Ager

Ages six to 11 are the elementary school years. Because kids grow and change very fast during this time, let's look at two periods: early and late stages.

Early School Age

In the early years, the school-age child is much like an older and more competent preschooler. The child is positive and curious and shows a great deal of initiative. The child attacks a task for the pure joy of being on the move in trying out what the world has to offer. The early school-age child is positive in his or her energy. If all goes well for the child, he or she will no longer have the toddler's need to protest independence. These kids are out to learn from parents, teachers, and friends. Preschoolers and early school-age children work hard at identifying, primarily with their same-sex parent, but also with both parents. Children of this age persist in stereotyped views of male and female roles, even if their parents avoid the stereotypes. Most of the time, children of this age will feel good about themselves and competent. At other times however, they will feel not so competent and will easily become discouraged as they become aware of the discrepancy between their own abilities and those of other children, especially older children.

The five- to seven-year-old stands at the crossroads between initiative and guilt. If the kids are provided with suitable opportunities, and successfully steered away from what is not suitable, they can come out of this period with a positive view of themselves while enjoying what the world has to offer. If, however, they are repeatedly allowed to fall into situations that will hurt or hinder their self-esteem, they can suffer tremendous emotional trauma. They can begin to fear challenges and attempts that would normally increase their confidence. A child's confidence is something that we never want to negatively affect—it is really the core and foundation to creating a healthy and successful child.

Late School Age

The late school-age period ranges from ages seven or eight onward, when the child begins to harness his or her personal drives and initiative. He or she begins to really explore everything in the environment. The child of this age group becomes more diligent and systematic about pursuing a task, and understands the useful purpose of creating something of value. By this age, children become more persistent and are no longer easily distracted. They also become better able to evaluate themselves once a task is completed. Kids at this age also value being independent from their parents and take pride in completing a task. Children at this age dislike being closely supervised, because they think they know more than their parents.

They want to develop self-control, so this is a good time to give them an opportunity to learn how to control their portions naturally, as a normal part of eating. The most effective technique for this is allowing kids to serve themselves the portion of food that they want. T Let them have more if they still seem to be hungry, but don't scold if they leave some food over. Insisting on a clean plate teaches kids to eat more even if they're not hungry, which often leads to weight problems later on.

School-age kids are quite capable of testing their limits. There will be times when they will be angry with you and put a lot of pressure on you. It's important for parents to stand their ground and not be intimidated by a child's outrage. Some parents avoid confrontation, but that is not an effective approach. It is much better to accept confrontation and to negotiate fairly with the child. This method will yield greater success. It may once again seem as if I'm off the point of childhood obesity, but I'm not really. Every bit of success with your child begins with understanding the mechanics of the psychology.

Presenting school-aged children with achievable tasks is a great way to build their confidence. Throughout history and even in some cultures today, young children contribute to their families by doing important work, such as helping with younger children, helping around the house, and helping with farm tasks. When kids are given age-appropriate responsibilities, they mature more quickly and have greater confidence in their own abilities. The benefit of this is that the adults begin to acknowledge the child as a valuable individual capable of making his or her own decisions. This process helps the child's confidence, which then leads to so many other positives, such as responsible eating and exercise. Parents need to really be hands-on throughout this developmental stage. If they are, and give praise for accomplishments and improvements, the chances of their child developing obesity or low self-esteem are much reduced. For children and adults alike, it is so important to be happy within ourselves, because happiness brings success. If a child isn't happy, he or she may unconsciously overeat and develop a cushion of fat around the body, a sort of protective shell. Seeing kids being overweight and depressed is extremely difficult. Parents often avoid saying no to anything that the child asks for fear of hurting the child even more. This is a wrong approach. Even though the child may be depressed, parents must not validate behavior that is unacceptable. They need to seek out the reason for the depression—conflict with a teacher, a fight with a friend, family issues such as divorce—and help the child with his feelings.

Children also benefit from a strong network of friends to increase their feelings of self-worth. When friends get together or play or do something, all the kids enhance their social skills. Being part of a group of kids who get together a lot strengthen their confidence because they feel accepted. Also, kids are always in some sort of competition with one another, which also helps build confidence. It gives kids a feeling of competence when they can keep up with or even exceed what the other kids do. Of course, you want them to be competing over positive things, like who can run furthest, and not negative things, like who can eat the most candy or pick on the littlest kid the most. Adult supervision is important. This the age when self-esteem begins to develop. Along with a solid workout and diet regimen, healthy mental development will take place.

At this age, your kids shouldn't need any nutritional supplements beyond a regular multivitamin with minerals. A parent's role in preparing healthy meals is of the utmost importance. If the meals are healthy and well-balanced, your kid won't need any supplements. On the opposite end of the spectrum are the numerous chemical additives in processed foods that should be avoided by all means. Never could I stress enough to you the importance of eating foods that are either organic or locally farmed or raised, including fish that is wild caught. It's also important to choose foods that are low in salt and added sugar and have a minimal amount of ingredients in the contents. For example, when you are food shopping, always read the contents of the product. Let's look at a can of beans, for example. When you look at the ingredients list on the label, you will see the words beans, water, and possibly also salt. If there's anything else, such as preservatives, should look for another brand. That is it! By keeping it simple, and eating a product with minimal added ingredients, you are reducing the amount of chemicals that enter your body. You also avoid eating something that you could be allergic to, such as MSG, or that may cause water retention from added salt. Avoid harmful food additives and keep the amount of chemicals that enter your body to a minimum.

Harmful Food Additives
Artificial Colors
102 tartrazine
104 quinoline
107 yellow
110 sunset yellow

122 carmoisine

123 amaranth

124 ponceau

127 erythrosine

129 allura red

132 indigotine

133 brilliant blue

142 food green

143 fast green

151 brilliant black

155 chocolate brown

Flavor Enhancers

620-625 glutamates, MSG, HVP, HPP

627 disodium guanylate

631 disodium insinate

635 ribonucleotides

Preservatives

200-203 sorbic acid and sorbates

210-213 benzoic acid and benzoates

220-228 sulphur dioxide and sulphites

249-252 nitrates, nitrites

280-283 propionic acid and propionates

Antioxidants

310-313 gallates

319 TBHQ

320 BHA

321 BHT

Natural Color
160b annatto

Others
trans fatty acids
hydrogenated fats/oils
calcium proprionate

The School-Ager Diet

Parents should educate themselves in about nutrition because you need a lot of good information to give your kids the maximum benefits from the food they consume. Parents often make the mistake of relying on their children to eat the so-called "healthy" meals from the school cafeteria. This is definitely a mistake. The school cafeteria's first concern is staying within its budget, its second priority is for the food to taste good so the kids will eat it, and the third priority, much more distant priority is for the food to be nutritious. Yes, there are nutritional guidelines the school needs to follow, but these are followed to the bare minimum. The guidelines are also very distorted. Potato chips count as a vegetable, chocolate milk or sweetened yogurt as a dairy serving, and cookies made with some whole wheat as a grain serving. Nutritional requirements observed at a bare minimum result in your body's performance operating at a bare minimum. Why would you ever want to simply survive instead of thrive? Why would you want your kids to just barely do enough work in school to pass instead of getting straight A's? Why would you want your children to barely make it onto the baseball team instead of trying to be the star player? It's all about giving and receiving, 100 percent. Life is too short, and youth is even shorter. So why not do your best for your kid? Don't you want your child to perform at full potential? If you know that some simple changes would help your child perform at that next level, wouldn't you make them? A simple change in diet isn't too much of a sacrifice, but many adults are scared of change due to their own insecurities, generally complacent attitude, and fears of trying new methods. These inherent flaws will cause people to miss out on so many other opportunities. Only wise people can change their ways. Remember, all of you parents out there can make a huge change for the better in your children's performance. All it takes is a well-balanced meal plan for the family. Feeding your kids a proper breakfast, lunch, and dinner along with a few snacks will make a tremendous positive impact on their lives. You'll see changes for the better in their school performance, mood, and appearance.

In the chart below I show you a day of healthy eating for a normal school-age child. Look it over—you'll see that it's not that hard to give your child good nutrition.

Healthy Meal Day for the School-Ager

Breakfast	toasted high-fiber English muffin with low-fat cottage cheese and high-fiber, sugar-free fruit spread
Snack	raisins mixed with nonfat plain Greek yogurt
Lunch	light tuna in water mixed with raw vegetables and mustard on high-fiber rye bread
Snack	1 banana
Dinner	broiled salmon
	baked sweet potato
	steamed vegetables or salad
	sugar-free pistachio pudding made with skim milk
Snack	almonds

The School-Ager Workout

Kids at this age begin to develop muscularly as well. Suddenly small changes in their bodies begin to become evident. Sudden growth spurts begin to become the norm. Now that your child's body is well-nourished, we can begin a more intense workout regimen.

The school-ager's exercise routine should consist of two parts: cardiovascular and muscle-building. Cardiovascular training includes playing sports, running, riding a bicycle, swimming, gymnastics, dance, and other activities that involve running and moving. Muscle-strengthening workouts include push-ups, pull-ups, weight training and any other resistance exercises.

Activities for School-Agers

Cardio Routine

Team and individual sports	1 hour per day
or	
Running, bicycling, swimming, or similar activities	1 hour per day

Five-Day Muscle-Building Routine

Day 1: chest, shoulders, back
5 sets push-ups
5 sets pull-ups
Day 2: legs
5 sets free squats
5 sets walking lunges
5 sets standing calf raises
Day 3: chest, shoulders, back
5 sets push-ups
10 sit-ups
5 sets Indian push-ups
Day 4: legs
5 sets body squats
5 sets lunges
5 sets standing calf raises
Day 5: chest, back, shoulders
5 sets push-ups
5 sets pull-ups
50 crunches

Programs for the School-Ager

Developing a child into a physically strong and fit individual is most definitely a step in the right direction for his overall health and quality of life. For sure, when I was a school-aged child, never did I think of the term quality of life. At that age life is so innocent and beautiful. But even if I never thought of the quality of life aspect while growing up, that doesn't mean that it didn't exist. For kids, quality of life starts with not being overweight. The school-aged child also identifies and thrives at trying to be different from peers. Being different for girls and boys very commonly means being popular by being a good athlete. The most effective way that a child avoids depression, obesity, and other problems is by building self-esteem and confidence. Confidence is developed slowly in a child when goals are met and they receive positive reinforcement from parents. Simply believing in your child renders extremely positive results.

I am a very strong advocate for kids being involved in activity programs. Programs doesn't have to mean sports. Instead, it should a supervised activity that interests your child—it could be sports, it could be art, it could be the reading club at the library, it could joining the Boy Scouts. What's important is that your child enjoys it. Parents should do the research necessary in order to locate and evaluate a particular program that complements the child's natural talents and areas of interest. For example, if you see that your child loves to play with crayons and paint pictures, then you should look into an art program. The same follows for a child that loves sewing, soccer, dancing, reading, nature study, or whatever. Remember that a child's interest and passion can seem unusual to an adult, or might not be what you had hoped for your child. Never should the parent react negatively to the child's interest by saying, for example, "Painting is stupid!" or "Art is for girls, not boys." Rather, a good reinforcing response might be: "Wow! Painting! That's a great idea. I know you'll be good at it."

5: The Teenage Years

As your kid enters the teenage years, his or her body undergoes substantial changes through a big increase in sex hormones. The changes are both physical and emotional. For boys, the male hormone testosterone begins to skyrocket to extremely high levels. It brings about many masculine traits, including rapid growth, sexual maturity, facial hair, and a deeper voice, along with increased aggression, libido, and energy. Testosterone also increases the body's metabolism, which is why teenage boys are always hungry and can eat huge amounts of food without gaining weight.

Teenage girls experience a small rise in their testosterone levels, but at this age they are now primarily producing the female hormone estrogen. At this age, a young woman develops breasts, menstruates, grows taller, and becomes sexually mature.

Understanding the endocrine (hormone) system is very important in order to understand the mechanics of the body. You must understand the engine and its components in order to operate the moving machine properly. Teenagers mature at different rates, some much earlier or later than others. Careful attention must be paid to the teenager who matures late, because he or she is more likely to develop feelings of insecurity and lack self-confidence. Late bloomers get teased by peers and often feel self-conscious and less competent. Parents need to notice this and be very supportive. Negative feedback from the parents will only hinder the growth of self-esteem and confidence. Parents shouldn't joke about a kid's size or rate of growth.

Teenagers and parents must definitely take advantage of this era in the teenager's life because it will only last for a few years. Now is the time to encourage good eating habits, regular exercise, and focus on schoolwork.

Teenage boys need to train harder and eat more than their female counterparts. With proper nutrition and eating, you can avoid the negative side effects of certain foods, such as insomnia and water retention. Food such as monounsaturated fats (olive oil) will increase testosterone levels, as will polyunsaturated fats (omega-3 fish oils, lean meat, egg yolks, and nuts). Foods that can induce sleep because they are high in the amino acid tryptophan include bananas, lean turkey breast and milk. Foods that decrease water retention include vegetables and other high-fiber foods.

Foods for Hormonal Efficiency

To increase strength levels for teenagers:
> broiled fatty fish such as mackerel, sardines, and salmon and herring
>
> lean red meat such as London broil, eye round and ground round
>
> nuts such as almonds, walnuts, cashews, and peanuts
>
> oils such as extra virgin olive oil and canola oil
>
> fruits such as coconuts and avocados

Foods that induce deep sleep:
> milk and dairy products
>
> skinless turkey breast
>
> bananas

Foods that reduce water retention:
> drinking two to four quarts of water daily
>
> all vegetables
>
> low-salt diet
>
> whole foods with no additives

Foods that provide instant energy:
> fruits

Foods that provide sustained energy:

  whole-grain pasta

   brown or wild rice

  sweet potatoes

  old-fashioned oatmeal

Foods that build muscle:

  lean proteins

  skinless turkey and chicken breast

  lean red meat

  egg whites

  fish

  whey protein isolate (women) and soy protein isolate (men)

Foods that improve digestion:

  vegetables

  fruits

  wheat bran

  oat bran

  barley

Foods that improve the skin:

  two to four quarts of water daily

  olive oil

  fish

  foods rich in vitamins E and C

  egg yolks

Foods that quickly replenish the body after exercising:

  fruit

  skim milk

  brown sugar

  honey

Foods that lower blood pressure:

  vegetables

  fruit

old-fashioned oatmeal

fish

olive oil

Foods that lower cholesterol:

olive oil

almonds

walnuts

fish

old-fashioned oatmeal

vegetables

wheat bran

oat bran

Foods that improve cognitive function:

olive oil

canola oil

almonds

walnuts

fish

seaweed

flaxseed

Feeding Teens

I vividly remember when I was a teenager and how I exercised and ate. My training and meal regimen definitely wasn't the best. My parents were excellent cooks and our family meals were great. I was already an athlete, however, and from that perspective my family meals weren't the best. I was on the wrestling team and needed to lose weight without losing muscle. My family meals were nutritious, but, like most people, they would sacrifice nutrition by adding unwanted calories in order to improve the taste. Parents aren't perfect.

Sticking to a healthy diet is important, especially for athletes. It should be a long-term lifestyle, rather than a short-term one. I'm a strong advocate of making the diet fun and diversified so it's easier to follow over the long run. I've seen diet fads come and go. I've even tried some myself throughout the years.

I have seen what works in healthy eating, and that is to keep the diet interesting and fun. You have to stick with it a solid, slow and steady pace for it to be easy to follow for a long time. The results you want for your body are based on your diet. Everything from improved appearance to improved performance depends on what you eat. These results do not happen overnight. Why not construct a meal plan and exercise routine that can more easily be followed? Remember that this is a lifestyle. The sooner the teenagers realize this, the better and more successful their results.

Teen Diet Suggestions

These recommendations are for a normal-weight teenager. Always drink plenty of water each day.

Breakfast	flavored sugar-free oatmeal
	2/3 cup scrambled egg whites
	banana
Snack	high-fiber protein bar
Lunch	low-sodium turkey breast sandwich with lettuce
	and mustard on whole-grainbread
Snack	low-fat cottage cheese with blackberries
Dinner	grilled fish with lemon and pepper
	wild rice
	green salad with pepper, olive oil, and vinegar
Snack	peanut butter and jelly sandwich on whole-wheat bread

These recommendations are for an underweight teenager. Always drink two to three quarts of of water each day.

Breakfast	3 whole omega-3 eggs
	2 high-fiber waffles with sugar-free syrup

	strawberries on top of the waffles
Snack	1 fruit
Lunch	cheeseburger made with lean ground beef, 1 slice low-fat cheese, lettuce, tomato, onion, mustard on a whole-grain, high-fiber bun
Snack	1 glass 2 percent milk
Dinner	broiled salmon with lemon and olive oil sweet potato with low-fat butter steamed broccoli with low-fat melted cheese on top
Snack	all-natural peanut butter on whole-grain bread

These recommendations are for an overweight teenager. Always drink plenty of water each day.

Breakfast	3/4 cup egg whites, scrambled 1 cup unprocessed wheat bran with blueberries or raspberries, low-fat milk
Snack	1 fresh fruit
Lunch	1 scoop whey protein powder blended with water, ice, and almonds
Snack	1 raw cucumber
Dinner	broiled filet of flounder with lemon and pepper steamed string beans with fresh tomato sauce small salad with olive oil and vinegar
Snack	1 glass skim milk

Exercise for Teens

Exercise is something that is necessary for growing teens, but recently, it seems to have been steadily neglected. Long gone are the days when the streets were packed with kids playing sports, engaging in activities, and socializing all hours of the day outside. It seemed then as if the kids couldn't wait to get outside and see their friends. Today's youth spend much more time indoors. They're much more computer-savvy but are much less athletic and much more likely to be overweight.

Most people think that obesity is a simple physical problem. This is untrue. Being overweight is really an emotional and mental problem. When a child is overweight, the parent interprets this as the child not being active enough or eating too much. This is only part of the problem. When a child is overweight, he or she is suffering and needs more attention to his or her emotional needs.

Excessive eating is an addiction; it provides instant gratification followed by longer-lasting guilt as the unwanted calories add pounds. Drugs and alcohol almost fall into this category, because those who suffer from drug and alcohol addiction also often suffer from depression or another mental illness. Addicts also seek instant gratification as a means to escape their feelings of pain and sadness. The drug or alcohol addict also feels that guilt and pain, once the euphoric feeling of the abused substance wears off.

Nevertheless an obese teenager is more than likely suffering just as much as an addict does. We may not realize the extent of the problem. Once again, the parents must really get involved by preparing healthy meals and helping the teen to be more physically active. Parents should try their hardest to prevent their children from getting to the point of being overweight. Chances are that by the time the teen is overweight, emotional problems have already begun to set in. The teenager can be so negatively affected that intervention might be needed to keep him or her from falling further into depression. Parents need to lead by example, by eating healthy meals and exercising with their children.

Exercise, of course, applies to everyone. Different teenagers will have different requirements, depending on their goals in fitness and whether or not they are competitive athletes, or overweight, or too thin. No matter what the need, there's a good, safe, and effective way to exercise.

If a teenager is overweight, he or she needs an exercise routine that requires more cardio. A teenager who is overweight but athletic may not need to diet; exercising regularly and playing sports may be enough to burn off the excess pounds. The activity doesn't have to be team sports, of course. Any low-impact, long-duration activity will help, such as dance class, martial arts, bike riding, or swimming. If the teenager is thin and not athletic, then weight training is an excellent option.

The activity that will yield the greatest results vary from teenager to teenager. That's why I use a method called meal and exercise customization. This entails devising meals and workout regimens that are made just for that particular individual. The choices are pretty much left to the teenager. He or she should get to choose the workouts and diets in order to feel more in control and more comfortable with the activity. Of course, they can only choose from selected healthy food choices and menu options, but that's OK. Teens also need some guidance, especially when it comes to nutrition. The choice of workouts is broader and lets the teen have more control.

Workouts for Teens

The workout below is a five-day resistance weight-training plan for an average teen who wants to get stronger and fitter. Ideally, the routine is done every day at about the same time. It's important to take the weekend off so the body can rest and recuperate. If the teen is already participating in an organized sports program, the plan may be adding too much exercise. Discuss it with the team coach or trainer first. If the teen's high school doesn't have a weight room, check out local gyms and YMCAs. The basic fees are usually affordable.

Monday: chest, abs

flat bench press	5 sets 12 repetitions
inclined dumbbell press	5 sets 10 repetitions
push-ups	2 sets 20 repetitions
crunches	50 repetitions

Tuesday: back, calves

pull-ups	5 sets 10 repetitions
lat machine pull-downs	5 sets 12 repetitions
dumbbell rows	2 sets 8 repetitions

Wednesday: shoulders, abs

lateral dumbbell raises	4 sets 15 repetitions
upright rows	4 sets 12 repetitions
front military press	4 sets 10 repetitions
leg raises	10 sets 10 repetitions

Thursday: biceps, triceps

straight bar curls	5 sets 10 repetitions
dumbbell curls	5 sets 12 repetitions
lying triceps extension	5 sets 10 repetitions
cable push-downs	5 sets 12 repetitions

Friday: legs, calves

squats	5 sets 10 repetitions
lunges	5 sets 12 repetitions
leg curls	5 sets 15 repetitions
standing calf raises	5 sets 25 repetitions

Cardio Plan for Teen Athletes

Early morning run	2 miles
or	
Early morning sprints	20 sprints
or	
Spin class	30 minutes
or	
Running up and down stairs	20 minutes

Organized Sports

I like to see kids and teenagers participate in organized sports, for several reasons. Playing organized sports help all kids get into good shape physically while having fun. For teens, they help build added coordination and improved cognitive function. Simple jogging, riding a bicycle, and sprinting do not involve quick decision-making or a constant change in body motion, as do sports such as tennis, soccer, or basketball. Organized sports help bring physical coordination and mental sharpness to the next level, by requiring your body to move at all different physical output levels, and in different directions. While jogging or riding a bicycle, your body is moving only in one set direction and does only repetitive movements. Your body becomes accustomed to that particular motion, and eventually, your growth and improvements become stagnant. Your body needs the challenge of adapting to any type of exercise or stress. In organized sports, your body is performing at all different cardiovascular levels. When your body is moving all sorts of directions, your coordination is improving. For example, whenever you begin a new sport or activity, you tend to look rather clumsy. That is because the movements are foreign to your body—you're not used to them. As you continue to practice the new activity, you slowly but surely start performing in a more coordinated manner. With continued practice, you eventually begin looking and performing like an expert. Coordination is an earned talent.

6: Calories

Calories are how we measure the amount of energy in a food. The more calories a food has, the more energy-dense it is and the more energy it provides. However, all calories are not created equal. Calories from junk food are often called empty calories, because they provide energy from low-value ingredients such as refined white flour and sugar. They don't provide any other nutritional value—no fiber, no vitamins, no other important nutrients. Today, most people get about a third of their daily calories—between 500 and 1800 calories a day—from junk food.

In general, you need to take in about 10 calories for every pound of your body weight just for your basic metabolism. So, if you weigh 150 pounds, you need a minimum of 1,500 calories a day. To that basic minimum, you need to add extra calories for your activity level. The usual way to calculate the extra calories is to multiply your weight by your activity level:

3 = sedentary
5 = moderate activity
7 = heavy activity
10 = intense activity

If you exercise moderately each day, determine your extra calorie needs by multiplying your body weight by 5. In our 150-pound example, that's another 750 calories a day, for a total of 2,250 calories. That amount of calories would make you feel energetic and able to get through your day and your workout. But if you take in much more than that without also increasing your activity level, you'll gain weight.

If you're overweight and take in fewer calories than you need to maintain your metabolism and your activity level, you will lose weight.

Why would you want to use your daily calories to consume foods that are empty of nutrition? These wasted calories come from cookies, sweets, and snack foods that do absolutely nothing positive for your body. On the contrary, these wasted calories actually drain your body of valuable nutrients and energy. Alcohol also produces wasted calories and hurts the body at the same time. A small daily glass of red wine may have some benefits for your heart health and it is also enjoyable and relaxing. Much more than that, however, doesn't benefit your health and could be harmful. Consuming high-quality fast, carbohydrates, and protein will improve the performance of your body and help you keep your weight where you want it.

When preparing family meals, you must first take into consideration nutritional requirements. These will vary, depending on your child's daily calorie expenditure, meaning how active your child is throughout the day. Think about your kid's current physical condition. Is he or she too heavy? Very strong or on the weak side? What are his or her physical goals? For example, if he is lifting weights or is very active in some other way (running cross country, for instance), his body will require more calories in the form of high-quality protein and carbohydrates. This is especially important for meals that follow workouts.

OK, I understand that kids are kids and they will always need to eat some junk food. Within limits, that's perfectly fine. When shopping for junk food, make the best of it by looking for the healthiest choices. Light popcorn, for instance, is a good choice; so is organic jerky. Sugar-free and low-fat versions of favorite treats aren't necessarily any better than the original versions. Often the low-fat versions have more added sugar to make up for missing fat; the sugar-free versions use artificial sweeteners.

When preparing meals, always include a green salad and a vegetable. The dietary fiber in greens, veggies, beans, and fruit are great for making you feel full on fewer calories, plus these foods are full of vitamins, minerals, and antioxidants. Usually a feeling of fullness is bad, because it most often means that you ate too much. But feeling full from lots of high-fiber vegetables isn't bad at all. Fiber is definitely the most overlooked and best-kept secret in the world of dieting. Its benefits go on and on. Another benefit of dietary fiber is that it acts like a broom in your intestines, moving things along and sweeping away waste products and bacteria. If you don't eat much fiber, you're likely to have digestive problems such as gas, bloating, and constipation. Waste products can build up in your intestines and give off toxins that make you ill—and this illness is called colon cancer. Scary, isn't it? The good news is that colon cancer may be avoidable if you eat a proper diet high in fiber.

Fiber is made up of the indigestible parts of plant foods; fiber is what give celery its crunch. It occurs naturally comes in two forms: soluble and insoluble. Soluble fiber dissolves, absorbs water, and forms bulk as your food moves through your intestines. Soluble fiber is found in fruit and oatmeal, among other sources. Insoluble fiber doesn't dissolve but rather carries waste along. Both are necessary and beneficial. In general, nutritional experts recommend that adults should get 25 to 30 grams of fiber a day; the average American gets less than 15 grams. Toddlers should get about 19 grams of fiber per day; older kids need about 25 grams. Starting at around age 9, kids should be getting at least 25 grams a day.

Processed foods, refined foods, fast food, and other manufactured foods are very low in fiber. The best way to get plenty of fiber in your diet is to swap candy bars, junk food, white bread, and other manufactured foods for whole, unprocessed foods whenever possible. Eat plenty of whole grains, vegetables, and fruit. When food shopping, look for the words "high-fiber" on the produce. Always read the food label, looking for the highest fiber content possible. For example, use brown rice instead of white and whole-wheat pasta instead of semolina pasta.

High-Fiber Foods

The best way to add fiber to the diet is by eating more salad, fruits, vegetables, whole-grains, nuts, and beans as part of your normal daily meals. Bran cereals and high-fiber versions of favorite foods can also help. Although it's always best to get fiber from your food, fiber supplements such as Nosy, Metamucil, and fiber pills and mixes can be used.

Breakfast	high-fiber pancake mix
	Fiber One high-fiber cereal
	old-fashioned or steel-cut oatmeal
	unprocessed wheat bran
	oat bran
	high-fiber whole-grain toast
	high-fiber English muffins
Snacks	fruits such as figs, raspberries, blueberries, blackberries, apples, pears
	nuts
	high-fiber protein bars
	Fiber One muffin mix
Lunch	whole-grain pita bread
	high-fiber wraps
	vegetables of all sorts
Dinner	sweet potato
	brown or wild rice
	whole-grain pasta
	salads
	vegetables of all sort

7: Desserts and Sweets

A lot of people think of healthy eating or dieting as a major sacrifice that doesn't allow for sweets, desserts, or any sort of treat. This isn't true at all! If you understand nutrition, you know how to choose wisely and can easily enjoy dessert and special treats.

Sugar Crashes

But first, let's talk about why you have to choose desserts wisely. When you eat a lot of sugar all at once, as happens when you eat, for example, a big piece of chocolate cake with icing, you can end up having a bad sugar crash. Here's how it happens: You eat the cake and send a lot of sugar into your system. Your blood glucose skyrockets, so your pancreas produces extra insulin to carry it off to be stored as fat. But when you overload your system with a big dose of sugar, your pancreas can overshoot the target and carry off more glucose than it should. That actually drops your blood sugar too low—you get a sugar crash. The crash is called hypoglycemia. The usual symptoms of hypoglycemia are feeling shaky, spaced out, tired, and suddenly very hungry for something sweet. The craving is your body's reaction to low blood sugar—it makes you want to eat something with a lot of carbohydrates to bring your blood sugar back up to normal. This roller-coaster experience is something that you definitely want to avoid at all costs.

During my early years of dieting, sugar crashes were a tremendous obstacle for me to overcome. Because I didn't know any better, sugar highs and lows became a vicious cycle for me. While I was depriving my body of complex and fibrous carbohydrates, my energy levels would decrease. Then I would drink coffee in order to increase my energy and compensate. Eventually, I would become immune to the caffeine and would become tired again. In addition, because my body was being deprived of carbohydrates, it would crave sugar. By the time I ate carbs at the end of the day, my energy levels would spike, then crash all of a sudden again, because sugars only provide very short-term energy. Basically, I was putting my body on a seesaw ride by making my energy and mood go up and down all day long. This is really the hard way to diet.

Through nutrition study and trial and error, over the years I have developed a much more effective method of dieting. It lets me look lean while still eating some sweets. You, too, can have your cake and eat it.

Good Dessert Choices

Always look for the healthiest alternatives, such as fresh fruit, sugar-free gelatin, sugar-free pudding, and plain Greek yogurt (top the yogurt with berries and other fruit for sweetness).

Here's a list of tasty, low-calorie dessert options that I enjoy:
• Fresh fruit (any kind you like)
• Sugar-free, fat-free puddings: these come in lots of great flavors, including pistachio, chocolate, vanilla, fudge, cheesecake, tapioca, and strawberry
• Sugar-free, fat-free gelatin: these also come in great flavors, including orange, blackberry, lemon, cherry, lime, strawberry, and kiwi. Gelatin is very quick and easy to prepare.
• Sugar-free, fat-free frozen yogurts
• Sugar-free, fat-free ice cream
• Sugar-free, fat-free whipped cream
• Sugar-free, fat-free cakes
• Sugar-free, fat-free rice pudding (made with brown rice, skim milk and sweetened with stevia)

Here are some dessert ideas:
- A cup of blueberries and/or strawberries with topped with whipped cream
- Sugar-free, high-fiber waffle topped with whipped cream
- Pudding topped with whipped cream and almonds
- Fat-free, sugar-free cheesecake topped with whipped cream and strawberries
- Milkshake made with fat-free, sugar-free ice cream, skim milk and blueberries
- Ice cream sundae made with fat-free, sugar-free fr oz.en yogurt, whipped cream, and raspberries
- Fat-free, sugar-free pumpkin pie
- Protein shake made with cookies and cream fat-free ice-cream, whey protein, and all natural peanut butter
- Protein pudding made with chocolate-flavored whey protein isolate, blended with water until very thick, then refrigerated and served dusted with cinnamon
- Fruit smoothie made with fresh fruit blended with ice
- Sorbet made with fresh strawberries, blueberries, blended and fr ozen

Sugar

I cannot stress to you enough the importance of satisfying your sweet tooth without eating sugar in its many versions. Sugar is a healthy person's worst enemy. Natural sweeteners such as white (table) sugar, brown sugar, high-fructose corn syrup, honey, and maple syrup really must be avoided at all costs when engaging in a healthy meal plan. Today, it's easier than ever to avoid sugar because there are so many artificial sweeteners that taste as good without the calories. Even so, it's important to break away from consuming very sweet foods and drinks. Regardless of whether they are natural or artificial, sweeteners cause your body to develop a dependence and tolerance. Eventually, you need more and more sweetness. After a while, when you drink a cup of coffee with sugar or sweetener in it, for instance, it will seem less sweet. You'll then start adding more sweetener. Even if you use a zero-calorie sweetener, it is still negatively affecting you: eventually you lose a sense of taste for the coffee. Too much sweetness will completely alter the taste of the food itself.

The other major drawback to having any type of sweetener is that your body begins to develop a tolerance toward anything sweet. What eventually happens is you begin to crave sweets more and more, to the point where you could be thinking about sweets all day long. It's definitely wise to limit your sugar and opt for the zero-calorie substitute.

Another factor that you must always take into consideration is that many sweetened products claim that the product is made with "all-natural sweetener" and is "sugar-free." What this really means is that actual white sugar may not be added, but other natural sugars are added instead, such as high-fructose corn syrup. These sweeteners are just as bad as sugar.

Sugar has too many negative drawbacks. For example, it causes premature aging because it combines with protein (glycated) in your body. As an example, think of the French dessert crème brûlée. This dessert is a custard topped with sugar that is heated under the broiler or with a kitchen torch to caramelize it. Exactly the same thing can happen inside your body when you have too much sugar in your bloodstream. Keep your sugar intake to a minimum by having sweets only once in a while.

Another negative drawback to having sugar is the increased appetite you will have shortly after eating it. After the energy-increasing effects wear off, you become hungry again, which makes you end up consuming more calories. Sugar also causes sleepiness, usually about an hour after it is ingested in quantity. For example, have you ever felt sleepy after eating a large meal? That is because you either ate too much sugar or fast-acting carbohydrates (or both).

Sugar and Artificial Sweeteners

Sugar is hidden in many manufactured food products, even including soups and salad dressings. To find it, look on the ingredients list for sugar under its many different names:

cane sugar

dextrose

glucose

sucrose

raw sugar

cane syrup

high-fructose corn syrup

corn syrup

sugar

maltose

lactose

fruit concentrate

Instead of adding sugar, try these natural sweeteners:

applesauce

yogurt

honey

fresh fruit

fresh fruit preserves, jellies and jams

fruit juice

Low- or zero-calorie artificial sweeteners include:

sucralose (Splenda)

saccharin (Sweet'N Low)

stevia

luo han guo

aspartame (NutraSweet, Equal)

8: Carbohydrates

Carbohydrates comprise one of the three main food groups, along with fat and protein. They provide the energy necessary to fuel the body. They fall into two basic categories, in terms of how quickly they enter your body in the form of glucose. Simple carbohydrates are quickly digested and enter your body quickly; complex carbohydrates are digested more slowly and enter your body slowly.

Knowing which carbohydrates to eat and when to eat them is really the secret to success for having a nice body that is lean, toned, and full of energy. Simple carbohydrates both enter and leave your system rapidly. The best time to ingest them is when your body is empty of food, and no sugar is in the bloodstream. These times typically occur either first thing in the morning after you've been asleep for hours, or right after exercising. At these two points, your body is drained of nutrients and needs energy put into its system rapidly.

Foods that are considered simple carbohydrates include fruits, sugar and honey. Refined foods, such as bread, pasta, and white rice are also digested quickly. For breakfast when you need quick energy, a good choice would be whole-wheat toast with honey, preserves, or fresh fruit. After a workout the same applies, but the choice in your foods usually changes. Right after a workout, a tablespoon of honey or some sugary fruit (such as watermelon or an orange) will work great to replenish your body's natural sugar.

Foods that are very low in fiber because they have been refined or processed also qualify as fast-burning carbohydrates. Fat and fiber tend to slow down the food's absorption rate, limit eating these foods to breakfast or right after training. If you don't eat some fast-acting carbs to replenish yourself after a workout, your body may begin to consume its own muscle tissue for food (cannibalization). To avoid this, it's very important never to skip those meals.

Dieters almost always make the mistake of skipping meals in order to lose weight. This never works, ever. Skipping meals slows down your metabolism which, in turn, makes your body burn fewer calories to adjust to the reduced calorie intake. Also, skipping meals makes you feel hungry, so you're likely to make up the calories you skipped when you have your next meal.

When losing body fat, the goal is to speed up your body's metabolism so your body will burn more calories throughout the day. Another common mistake is failing to eat the proper foods immediately following exercise. Right after a workout, your body craves carbohydrates and protein to replenish sugars and repair muscle tissue damage from resistance exercise. Your post-workout meal is by far the athlete's most important meal of the day. After working out is when your body really needs all the nutrients that it can get. Immediately following a workout, the most important food to have is a small amount of a simple carbohydrate, such as fruit or honey, to provide the instant energy that your body needs. The sugar will spike your insulin levels, which will provide the transport of nutrients to the rest of the body. Normally, it's best not to consume too many simple carbohydrates at one time. You need the fast-acting energy, but any carbs that you don't use right away will turn to fat. In the long-term, eating too much sugar and refined carbohydrates can lead to type 2 diabetes.

Measured in grams, a good post-workout meal or breakfast serving should be approximately 30 to 40 grams of carbohydrates. This is about the amount in one piece of fresh fruit or two tablespoons of honey. This may not seem like a large enough portion, but this is only in addition to your regular meal.

Simple Carbohydrates

Simple, fast-acting carbohydrates include sugar, fresh fruit, honey, fruit juice, fruit jelly and preserves, fructose, sucrose, corn syrup, fruit concentrate. Of these, your healthiest choices are fresh fruit or honey.

Breakfast and Post-Workout Meals with Added Simple Carbohydrates

2 whole eggs and 1/2 cup of oatmeal with honey

3/4 cup scrambled egg whites, 1 banana, and high-fiber bran cereal

1 1/2 cups whey protein isolate blended with 8 almonds, strawberries, and 1/3 cup nonfat Greek yogurt

6 oz. London broil with 1 cup brown rice, green salad, watermelon

Many different meal choices make perfect post-workout or breakfast meals. Choose the meal options that work best for you, because this healthy lifestyle is really for the long run. The easier the diet is to follow, the easier it will be for you to achieve your results.

Most of these very nutritious meals are not served at the school cafeteria. A teenager needs to make the necessary adjustments by choosing the best foods from what's available—fruit, for instance, is almost always available. Overall, however, it's probably better for a teenager to bring his own properly prepared food from home.

Better Carbohydrates

Some carbohydrates fall right in the middle between fast-acting and slow-acting. They should be avoided because they are not as fast-acting as simple carbohydrates nor do they provide the fiber of the complex carbohydrates. In other words, there are so many better choices of carbohydrates that you can eat. These include bran cereals with added sugar, white rice, white potatoes, white pasta, and white bread. To avoid the problem with these carbohydrates, choose them in the slower-acting whole-grain versions instead. Swap white potatoes for sweet potatoes.

Complex carbohydrates are slower-burning because they contain fiber. Complex carbohydrates provide a steady stream of energy for your body. Consuming the proper amount of them will provide your body with constant energy, but without the spikes and crashes that simple carbohydrates can cause. The proper serving size is, once again, dependent upon your kid's caloric expenditure and at what time of the day these foods are eaten. Consuming too many complex carbohydrates in one sitting will lead to gaining body fat and feeling tired after eating. It is important always to watch your portions. These carbohydrates burn slower because they also consist of fiber which is indigestible food. Whenever you are food shopping, always look for the words "high-fiber." Remember that sugar will always speed up digestion when added to food, while fiber will slow down the digestion.

Good Complex Carbohydrates

Good complex carbohydrate choices are made from unrefined foods. The portion size should be between 30 and 50 grams (about half a cup), depending on the person's weight, caloric expenditure, and the time of the day that the food is consumed.

sweet potatoes

yams

brown rice

old-fashioned oatmeal

oat bran

wheat bran

whole-grain pasta

vegetables

wild rice

quinoa

kashi

whole-grain bread

whole-grain wheat bran

9: Fiber

Fiber is such an overlooked aspect of nutrition. Fiber has no nutritional value, no vitamins, and no nutrients but it is extremely valuable as part of your food. Fiber is the indigestible part of plant foods, such as the cellulose that forms cell walls and make carrots crunchy. Fiber comes in two forms: soluble and insoluble. Soluble fiber absorbs water while insoluble does not. In other words, as soluble fiber passes through your system it expands and becomes bulkier because the soluble fiber is absorbing water along the way. While expanding, it acts as an intestinal cleaner and absorbs excess fluids to be carried out of your body. While insoluble fiber does not dilute in water, it passes through your intestines more rapidly, carrying waste products along.

Fiber adds a sense of fullness to your meal while maintaining a healthy digestive system. It's not necessary to get too technical about the two different fibers—in natural foods such as fruits and vegetables, you get plenty of both.

Another benefit of eating enough daily fiber (25 to 50 grams a day) is that it reduces the chances of getting colon cancer. Colon cancer begins to be diagnosed usually after the age of forty, because most people neglect their fiber intake their entire lives. After years of undigested food accumulation in the intestines, the decaying organic matter begins to cause damage and illness to the intestines, which then can lead to cancer. Simply increasing your fiber intake will reduce this drastically. Another benefit to consuming sufficient fiber is that it rids the intestines of undigested food, which in turn makes you a few pounds lighter. You will feel a lot more nimble as well. This is a refreshing and energetic feeling.

Fiber also has the tremendous advantage of making you feel full but without the guilty calories. This is my favorite benefit to eating fiber, because this advantage has helped me tremendously throughout the years. By eating a high-fiber diet I can keep my body fat at its lowest levels but without have to endure feelings of hunger. Years ago, when I knew less about nutrition, I would suffer quite a bit to stay in shape, because I was always hungry. But now, thanks to adding a lot more fiber to my diet, I no longer suffer uncomfortable bouts of hunger and food cravings.

Fiber is really a type of starch (carbohydrate) that our digestive system doesn't break down easily, so it passes on through without being digested. Fiber is found in fruits, vegetables, beans, nuts, and whole grains. It adds bulk to your diet and helps prevent constipation. Eating more fiber has endless benefits, including making you feel better and decreasing the risk of many diseases such as colon cancer, cardiovascular diseases, and diverticulitis. High-fiber foods tend to be more filling, so you feel satisfied after eating with fewer calories.

High-fiber foods are easy to add to your diet. All vegetables are good source, such as cabbage, kale, broccoli, all beans, and green beans. Fruits such as figs, blueberries, apples, raspberries, and blackberries are good options. At breakfast, try cereals such as unprocessed wheat bran, oat bran, and steel-cut oats.

When adding more fiber to your meals and snacks, start slowly and increase a little at a time. This allows your digestive system to adjust to the change. Increasing fiber too quickly can cause gas, bloating, and cramps. It is also important always to drink plenty of water because fiber, especially soluble fiber, expands with water and softens the food in your digestive tract, allowing for easier passage through your intestines.

High-Fiber Muffin Recipe
1 cup water
1 cup skim milk
1 cup raisins

1 cup rolled oats

1 1/4 cups traditional whole-wheat flour

1 1/2 cups unprocessed wheat bran

1 1/2 teaspoon baking soda

Preheat oven to 350 degrees F. Simmer raisins and water for 5 minutes and set aside to cool slightly. In large bowl, stir together dry ingredients. In a separate bowl, combine simmered water, raisins and milk. Stir the liquid ingredients into the dry ingredients, just barely combining. Scoop mixture into greased muffin tins or into a loaf pan. Bake muffins for 20 minutes; bake loaf for 1 hour or until toothpick comes out clean. Makes 12 muffins or 1 loaf.

High-Fiber Meals

The dinner portions for these meals are large to help you refuel after your workout. Be sure to drink lots of water throughout the day and especially after a workout (one quart).

Regular Meal

Breakfast	1 cup high-fiber toasted oat cereal with lactose-free skim milk 1/2 grapefruit
Snack	raw celery with low-fat cream cheese
Lunch	whole-grain macaroni and low-fat cheese with black pepper
Snack	high-fiber protein bar
Dinner	salad with nonfat feta cheese, lettuce, tomato, onion, extra virgin olive oil, balsamic vinegar with a few walnuts sprinkled on top 6 oz. broiled fish steamed vegetables with melted low-fat cheese 1 cup wild rice with onion 1 quart water
Dessert	sugar-free, fat-free cheesecake-flavored pudding

Vegan Meal

Breakfast	1 whole-grain, high-fiber English muffin with fruit preserves and all-natural peanut butter
	fresh fruit with almonds
Snack	1 banana
Lunch	1 cup Kashi cereal with lactose-free skim milk
	1 cup whole-grain pasta with fresh tomato sauce
	1 tablespoon almond butter
Dinner	extra-firm low-fat tofu served with vegetables sautéed in olive oil and garlic
	whole-grain bread
	sweet potato with non-dairy low-fat cream
	salad with almonds, walnuts, olive oil, vinegar

Vegetarian Meal

Breakfast	2 whole omega-3 eggs
	2 whole-grain, high-fiber pancakes with sugar-free syrup
	1 cup 100 percent fruit juice
Snack	light protein shake
Lunch	broiled fish sandwich with high-fiber rye bread, lettuce, onion, tomato, low-calorie tartar sauce
Dinner	1 steamed lobster and shrimp with garlic
	1 cup brown rice
	steamed Brussels sprouts with melted low-fat sharp cheese

10: Protein

Protein provides the building materials for all the cells in the body. The building materials are called amino acids, and there are twenty different ones that are essential to good health. Protein is used to grow tissue, bone, organs, and blood and to make the many hormones, antibodies, and enzymes that keep the body running properly. Protein can come from animals or from plants. Protein from animals (beef, poultry, fish, dairy products and eggs) is considered the best source because they are complete: they provide all the essential amino acids in the right proportions. No plant foods contain all the essential amino acids. To get a complete protein serving with all the essential amino acids from only plant foods, two or more need to be combined, such as beans and rice. Plant proteins include nuts, beans and lentils, corn, soy milk, and other soy products such as tofu. Beans contain six of the eight essential amino acids, brown rice contains a different set of five amino acids. There will be some overlap, but together they fill any gaps that the other food might be missing. These plant food combinations are found in many cultures. For Americans, it may be a peanut butter sandwich on whole-wheat bread. In Middle Eastern cultures, it could be lentils and rice. In Latino cultures, it may be rice and beans or corn tortillas and beans. In the Italian culture it is pasta with beans. All of these combinations are a healthy substitute for meat because they are less expensive, often have much less fat, and always have more fiber (meat does not have fiber).

Eating an adequate amount of protein has other advantages as well, such as the feeling of satiety. After eating protein you will always feel full. The difference with protein, as opposed to fats and especially carbohydrates, is that feeling of fullness doesn't mean getting fat, because protein is similar to fiber in giving that feeling of fullness that quickly goes away while your body still remains satisfied. Fiber is not a protein. Thus, by eating fiber alone, your body will not function properly. When eating protein, as it is digested it is used to repair and build muscle tissue, which is why it is so important to be active and lift weights if possible in order to constantly tear muscle tissue in your body that the protein will repair. Whenever you eat protein, especially after resistance training, the protein goes right to work repairing your muscle tissue that was productively torn during training.

Another reason eating a high-protein diet leads to less body fat is because your body burns more calories during the process of digesting protein. In other words, for every 100 calories of protein you eat, fewer calories are left to be used by your body or stored as fat, because the protein digestion process requires your body to work harder. When you eat 100 calories of protein, you may only absorb about 60 calories after it is digested. By contrast, carbohydrates are much easier to digest. When you eat 100 calories of carbohydrates,
your body will absorb 80 calories after digestion.

This all may seem a bit technical, but I'm giving you an in-depth explanation of why high-protein, high-fiber diets work best for fat loss, building muscle and strength, and overall health and well-being.

Lean Protein Recommendations

Portion size should be between 6 and 8 ounces before cooking. Choose organic and free-range, grass-fed products whenever possible. Local farmers' markets are a good source.

Beef cuts: top round (London broil), eye round, 93 percent ground lean

Chicken: skinless, boneless breast

Turkey: skinless, boneless breast

Pork: boneless loin

Fish: any wild-caught species

Seafood: lobster, crab, shrimp, octopus, shellfish

Game meat: buffalo, venison, duck, buffalo, wild boar, emu, ostrich
Eggs
Whey protein isolate
Soy protein isolate

Proteins with carbohydrates
Skim milk (lactose free)
nonfat Greek yogurt
nonfat cottage cheese
nonfat cheese

Daily Menus with High-Quality Protein
Standard High-Protein Diet
Note: Drink two to four quarts of water daily.

Breakfast	2 whole omega-3 farm-raised eggs
	1 Fiber One bran muffin
Snack	1 cup nonfat cottage cheese with blueberries
Lunch	light tuna in water mixed with nonfat mayonnaise and celery
Snack	2 tablespoons all-natural peanut butter
Dinner	hamburger made with 93% lean ground beef with whole-grain bun, lettuce, tomato, onion, mustard and ketchup
	sugar-free jello
Snack	low-fat cheese slices

Seafood Protein Diet
Note: Drink two to four quarts of water daily.

Breakfast	1/2 cup nonfat Greek yogurt
	1 toasted cinnamon bagel
	1 cup strawberries with nonfat whipped cream
Snack	2 tablespoons all-natural peanut butter

Lunch	sautéed shrimp with spinach, garlic, onion and brown rice
Snack	1 fruit
Dinner	steamed crab legs with melted butter
	steamed carrots with nonfat sour cream
	sweet potato
	sugar-free, nonfat ice cream
Snack	8 to 10 almonds

Fish Protein Diet
Note: Drink two to four quarts of water daily.

Breakfast	whey protein isolate blended with apple, oats, almonds, ice, water
Snack	1 cup nonfat Greek yogurt
Lunch	canned salmon mixed with broccoli and rice
Snack	apple, 1 tablespoon peanut butter
Dinner	broiled trout with white wine and onion
	whole-grain pasta with grated nonfat cheese
	salad with olives, feta cheese (nonfat), extra virgin olive oil, lemon, lettuce, onion, tomato, broccoli, and black pepper
	rice pudding made with stevia, cinnamon, skim milk and brown rice
Snack	low-fat cheese slices

11: Fats

At one time low-fat diets were recommended, but today you really don't hear too much about them. Although we associate eating fat with being fat, in reality low-fat diets or no-fat diets have never been shown to be very effective. For many years, however, the entire country seemed to believe in the low-fat theory for weight loss. People believed that eating fat would cause you to become fatter, so eating a lot less fat would make you become thinner. This concept turned out to be false. Food manufacturers benefited greatly by selling "low-fat" or " nonfat" foods, but the people eating these foods, especially kids and teenagers, kept getting heavier and heavier. The food industry thrived, and so did weight gain.

There are two main thoughts behind the low-fat diet concept. The first is that fat is the source of the extra calories kids and teenagers consume. Gram for gram, fat has more calories than carbohydrates and protein. Fat has nine calories per gram, while protein has four, as do carbohydrates. Foods that are high in fat tend to be more tasty. Who doesn't like fried chicken or potato chips or ice cream? Right? So kids and teenagers may eat more high-fat foods because they taste good. Saturated fat may contribute to heart attacks and strokes that occur from the increase in "bad" cholesterol and triglycerides. However, research has shown that eating fats does not necessarily lead to weight gain.

An extremely low-fat diet can cause problems of its own. Certain vitamins that your body requires, such as vitamin E and D, are known as fat-soluble vitamins, which means that they can only be absorbed into your body if they are eaten with fat. That's why it's a good idea to prepare vegetables with olive oil. This is also the main reason why salad is served with oil and vinegar dressing. Without the oil, the salad's vitamins will not be absorbed as well into the body. Another reason low-fat diets are unhealthy is because, without eating sufficient fats, your liver's enzymes begin to elevate to unhealthy high levels.

Fats are needed to help your body produce a number of important hormones, including testosterone. A study of athletes on the Ohio State University wrestling team looked at testosterone levels before and after the athletes went on a strict low-fat diet. Not surprisingly, the athlete's testosterone levels were a lot lower after they began their low-fat diets. And as we all know, testosterone is a necessary hormone, especially for sports, so we wouldn't want to lower it at any cost.

A healthy diet should be between 20 and 30 percent fat, but they need to be healthy fats such as olive oil and the natural fats in nuts. A healthy diet includes some healthy fats that are mono- or polyunsaturated. A diet rich in these fats, along with fiber-rich carbohydrates and lean proteins, leads to having a lean and strong body. Fats are powerhouse foods because they pack more calories per gram than protein or carbs. Fats keep us warm, make bodily processes work better, and taste good, too.

Types of Fat

Saturated fat	animal fat, butter, coconut oil
Monounsaturated fat	(almonds, cashews, peanuts, and pecans), avocado, olive oil, olives, canola oil, sesame seeds, peanut butter, peanut oil, grape seed oil, flaxseed oil
Polyunsaturated fat	corn oil, safflower oil, soybean oil, sunflower oil, walnuts, pumpkin seeds, sunflower seeds
Omega-3 fatty acids	walnuts, flaxseed, flaxseed oil, canola oil, albacore tuna, herring, mackerel, sardines, rainbow trout, salmon

One fat should be avoided at all costs: trans fat. Trans fats are created during a process called hydrogenation that is used to turn liquid vegetable oil into solid fats. A lot of research has shown that trans fat is much worse than saturated fat (butter) for cardiovascular risk. Manufacturers are now required to list the amount of trans fat per serving in the nutritional label. Look for none, or less than 0.5 mg per serving. Going forward, the FDA has decided that trans fats should not be used at all. Food manufacturers are gradually phasing them out.

Some typical foods containing trans fat are processed foods (cakes, crackers, chips, and cookies), some stick margarine, shortening, and some French fries. Avoid these always.

Healthy Meals with Good Fats

Menu 1

Breakfast	2 whole omega-3 eggs
	1/2 cup oat bran
	1 kiwi
Snack	8 to 10 almonds
Lunch	can of albacore tuna in olive oil with celery, onions on a whole-grain pita bread
Snack	all-natural peanut butter with 1 slice whole-wheat bread
Dinner	broiled salmon with onion and lemon
	butternut squash with olive oil
	salad with walnuts and olive oil
	1 cup lentils with all-natural butter
Snack	low-fat cheese slices

Menu 2

Breakfast	whey protein shake with walnuts, oats, pear
Snack	carrots with all-natural cream cheese
Lunch	light tuna with olive oil and pepper

	salad with feta cheese and olive oil, vinegar
Snack	2 tablespoons all-natural peanut butter
Dinner	broiled fish with lemon
	sweet potato with olive oil
	vegetables with avocado
Snack	1 cup nonfat Greek yogurt

Note: Whenever possible, purchase wild-caught fish, which have a high concentration of healthy omega-3 fatty acids.

How to Eat More Healthy Fat

If you aim for a healthy diet, the right amount of good fats will naturally fall into place. If you want to get more fat in your diet, however, here are a few pointers

• If there is heart disease in your family it is good to recognize the disease and limit the intake of saturated fats. Use olive oil for cooking at low heat; stop eating fried food; eat at home and grill, bake and steam your food; after the age of two, begin reducing the children's milk from whole to 2%, to 1% and then eventually to nonfat milk.

• Serve meat with plenty of vegetables to minimize the red meat's health risks.

• Make your own hamburger patties with extra-lean ground beef or turkey breast; serve on whole-wheat, high-fiber buns.

• Even if you don't have a heart disease risk in your family, it is still wise to always limit your intake of saturated and trans fats.

If you really want to eat deep-fried or other high-fat foods, you can! One day a week, plan to have a cheat day, where you and your family can eat anything you want. That way, you get to enjoy some favorite foods without undoing the good diet you've followed the rest of the week. A cheat day lets you enjoy family events, social events, and so on without having to watch what you eat. It doesn't have to be the same day each week, but you can have only one cheat day in any one week.

Skip the low-fat, reduced-fat, and fat-free manufactured foods (foods like apples are fat-free naturally). These foods have a long list of added sugars, chemicals, and additives that are used to replace the fat. None of these are really healthy. Instead, eat more naturally lower fat foods such as fruits, vegetables, beans and legumes and whole grains. Vary your fat intake by eating both monounsaturated fats and poly-unsaturated fats, meaning nuts, fish, avocado and olive oil. Whenever serving higher fat foods, be sure to make the portions smaller and include plenty of fiber such as fruits, vegetables and legumes. Try to keep the high-fat portion size to around three ounces. Fats from vegetables, nuts and seeds are much better for you than saturated animal fats. Whole grains also have very little healthy fat. Egg yolks were long considered to be unhealthy because they naturally contain cholesterol and saturated fat. However, eggs also have many positives, including mono-unsaturated fat and vitamin E. It's perfectly healthy to eat one or two whole eggs a day. However, buy either fresh eggs at your local farmer's market or organic, cage-free and free-range eggs. These eggs are high in omega-3 fatty acids. My family in Spain eats fresh eggs right from the chicken coop in their backyard and you can immediately see and taste the difference. The yolk is such a colorful orange! And the taste! You will taste the difference immediately!

Whole milk because is high in saturated fat. Fat-free milk should always be your choice. Look for the lactose-free version. As kids and teenagers age, their ability to absorb lactose, the sugar in milk, naturally diminishes. This can cause gas, cramps, bloating, and diarrhea. Lactose is also a sugar and should be avoided for that reason as well. Buy organic, hormone-free brands. Lactose-free milk is a great source of nutrients and protein for your family.

12: Calcium

In the United States, dairy foods are traditionally been an important source of the mineral calcium for children. Over the past several decades, the trend has been for children to drink less milk and more soda. One of the consequences of this has been that kids don't get enough calcium, especially children the ages of 9 and 18. Children need calcium for good bone growth, so the trend isn't a positive one! Children are growing, and it is during adolescence that bones reach their peak of highest density. Having good bone mass in childhood is the best way to avoid osteoporosis, a crippling disease caused by thin bones, in later life.

Dairy foods aren't the only place to get calcium, however, and other factors are involved in bone growth as well. Exercise is crucial. The more exercise, the better the bone growth. For your body to absorb and use calcium most efficiently, you also need vitamin D, the sunshine vitamin. Vitamin D deficiency, also known as rickets, used to be common before dairy products started being fortified with supplemental vitamin D in the 1920s. Although severe vitamin D deficiency is rare today, many kids still don't quite get enough. Vitamin D is a unique vitamin because, while we get some from food like the other vitamins, the primary source is your own body. When your skin is exposed to sunlight, you produce vitamin D. Five to 15 minutes of direct sun exposure per day, during the spring, summer and fall (using SPF 8 sunscreen or less) will provide adequate vitamin D to meet your needs and see you through the cold, dark winter months. Unfortunately, most of us aren't outdoors in the sunshine very much. We're indoors much of the day for much of the week. When we do go out, we often put on sunscreen to block the sun's rays. To be sure of getting enough vitamin D, it's also important to eat foods that are high in it..

Vitamin D isn't found naturally in many foods. It's found in fatty fish, egg yolks, butter, and beef liver. That's why milk and margarine are fortified with vitamin D. Dairy foods, such as yogurt and cheese aren't made with fortified milk, however, so they're not good sources of vitamin D. Today many doctors recommend taking a daily vitamin D supplement.

Calcium is found in many foods besides dairy products, but in small amounts per serving. You can see from the list below that your non-milk-drinking 12-year-old would have to eat a lot of spinach and beans to get all of the necessary calcium. Fortified drinks such as rice milk and orange juice can help, but at the cost of a lot of sugar. If your child doesn't eat enough dairy foods, make sure he or she gets lots of healthy greens, beans, and tofu (bean curd). Talk with your pediatrician about whether your child is getting enough calcium and if a supplement is needed.

The Nutrition in Milk

	Calories	Protein (g)	Fat (g)	Sugar (g)	Calcium (mg)
Whole milk	146	8	8	13	276
2%	122	8	4.8	12	285
1%	102	8	2.4	13	285
Fat-free	83	8	0	13	306
Chocolate	190	8	4.8	24	272

Calcium Requirements for Kids

1–3 years old	500 mg/day = 2 cups of milk
4–8 years old	800 mg/day = 3 cups of milk
9–18 years old	1,300 mg/day = 4–5 cups of milk

Nondairy Calcium Sources

Tofu	150 grams	347 mg
White beans	3/4 cup	119 mg
Navy beans	3/4 cup	93 mg
Pinto beans	3/4 cup	53 mg
Tahini	2 tbsp	130 mg
Almonds	1/4 cup	93 mg
Salmon, canned with bones	3 oz.	188 mg
Collards	1 cup	266 mg
Spinach	1 cup	245 mg
Rhubarb	1 cup	348 mg
Soy beans (edamame)	1 cup	261 mg
Kale	1 cup	179 mg
Okra,	1 cup	177 mg
Chinese cabbage (pak-choi)	1 cup	158 mg
Greens: turnip, beet, dandelion	1 cup	150 mg

Eating sufficient calcium is not only necessary but, with time and experience, you will be able to notice for yourself whenever your body is deficient in calcium or any other nutrient. Your body really is a "fine running machine," meaning that once you become completely aware of your body and its performance, you will begin to notice the slightest changes in its function and the way you feel. You will be able to fine-tune your diet and workouts to best fit your needs and the way you feel during that particular day. Really learning and knowing your body is a process that doesn't happen overnight but will happen, provided you make the effort to maintain your healthy lifestyle by consistently exercising and eating correctly. Remember that achieving maximum results and performance is not our short-term goal at all. Our overall goal is to feel better, little by little, every day. I have always stated that it's not about perfection, but rather, constant and steady improvement. As a child, you will notice that by living this healthy lifestyle of eating responsibly and exercising, you will only experience your life getting better and better because you will feel better, look better, and be more confident. These are priceless benefits that you will achieve, provided that you make the necessary sacrifices that most people can't seem to do. This will catapult your appearance, performance, and feeling of well-being to the next level! I truly believe in you, so you must believe in yourself!

13: Vitamins and Minerals

Vitamins and minerals are key to every process that takes place in your body. They work in partnership with other nutrients in your food. You get vitamins and minerals only from eating a wide variety of foods, in particular, from eating lots of vegetables, fruit and whole grains. Research shows that you can lower the risk of cancer by eating such foods. Vitamin supplements have not been shown to be as effective as natural foods. Food always has been the best natural medicine and source of nutrients. I like to eat a variety of vegetables to help make sure I get a variety of vitamins and minerals throughout the week. I also try to buy my vegetables when they are in season and from local farmer's markets. In-season and locally grown fruits and vegetables always taste better and pack more nutrients due to their freshness and lack of chemicals. Don't worry too much about buying vitamins and supplements. If you follow the meal plans in this book, chances are good that you will get all the vitamins and minerals you need from your food alone; you may not need to add any supplements.

A lot of people are under the impression that the more vitamins and supplements they take, the healthier and stronger they will be. This is not the case at all. The dark side of supplements is they are a multi-billion-dollar industry that is also almost entirely unregulated. Back in 1994, the Dietary Supplement Health and Education Act came into effect. The law basically limited restrictions on supplement manufacturers. As long as the product was a dietary aid and did not make any specific health claims on the product label or advertisement, the product would not have to pass FDA approval in order to be sold in stores. In other words, anyone can make any type of vitamin, supplement, or weight-loss product and sell it in stores. No licenses, FDA approval, or proven medical claims—nothing is needed for the product to be sold. What this means is that a vitamin company can produce a "weight loss" pill that may consist of nothing but caffeine, put a picture of a thin person on the label, and claim that the product "supports" weight loss, and sell it, without any clinical proof at all. In the advertisements for the product, the company will be have all sorts of testimonials from people claiming it worked wonders for them, but never mention any scientific studies.

My suggestion to you is to be careful every time you step foot in a vitamin store. Most of the products aren't what they claim to be—you won't receive the results that you had expected. The sales staff will try to sell you a lot of additional products, because that's what they're hired to do. In my nearly thirty years of experience in fitness and weight loss, I must admit that I have fallen prey to supplement hype. In my earlier years I was looking for shortcuts and believed all the sales pitches thrown at me. I definitely learned a lot from all of this. I don't want you to make the same mistakes.

Keep it simple by buying only the supplements that really work and relying on natural, home-cooked foods that provide the best possible nutrition. There are two supplements that I do buy and truly believe in: whey protein isolate and multivitamins with minerals. I usually have one multivitamin daily and one serving of whey protein daily as well. The whey protein provides me with fast-acting protein after I train. I blend it into a delicious shake that really satisfies my sweet tooth! It's like having a milkshake but without the guilt.

14: Nutritional Labels

In order to really monitor all the food that enters your body (which, by the way, is the best way to attain the healthiest body possible), you need to be able to read and completely understand the nutritional labels that are on each and every food product. Years ago, before I really began to get into eating right, never would I even look on the back of a food package to read the nutrition facts label and the ingredients list that are on the package. Like most people, whenever I shopped, my main priority was buying for taste, and then cost. Never would I consider the nutritional value of the food. It wasn't until I was fourteen years old that I actually began to diet, but only so I could lose seven pounds in order to wrestle in the lighter weight class, which was 101 pounds. At that point in my life is when it all began. First, I had purchased small booklets that outlined foods and their calories, so I could begin to calculate and measure the number of calories I was eating and what changes in my diet I needed to make in order to lose the seven pounds. I then began reading health and fitness magazines so I could learn more about the number of calories I was burning throughout the day and which activities burned how many calories. By the time I was a seventeen-year-old senior in high school, I had learned about how to lose weight without burning muscle tissue. I did it by learning how to read the food label.

How to Read the Label
A food package has a lot of information on it. The container has an ingredients list that tells you everything that's in the food. It also has a nutrition facts panel that tells you about the nutritional value of the food.

First look at the ingredients list. Ingredients are always in order from the ingredient that weighs the most to the one that weighs the least. This is a good way to get an idea of how healthy the food it. If the primary ingredient is bleached enriched white flour, the food is probably not a good choice; if the first ingredient is 100 percent whole wheat, it's a better option. The primary ingredients should be most of the label. If the label has a long list of ingredients that you can't pronounce, that often means it's full of preservatives, additives, and salt.

Next, look at the nutrition facts box. This can be a little confusing, because it packs a lot of information into a small space. The first item is the serving size and number of servings per container. Pay careful attention to this, because it can be misleading. The container might have two or more servings, but it's easy to think that the rest of the information is for the whole container, not just one serving.

Next, look at the calories per serving. You may see that a serving is 80 calories and eat the whole box, not realizing that there were nine servings in the box, so you actually ate 720 calories! The next item on the list is the fat content. Read this carefully to be sure the food doesn't have any trans fats and contains at most 1 to 2 grams of saturated fat per serving. Any other fats listed, such as mono or polyunsaturated fat, are fine. Then, look at the cholesterol content to make sure it's as close to zero as possible. Then check the sodium content; again, as close to zero as possible is healthiest. Then look at the total carbohydrates, which tells you a lot about the fiber and sugar content of the food. Finally, look at the protein. The rule of thumb here is the higher the better, but not to exceed 40 grams per serving. A balanced meal would be about 30 to 40 grams of protein, 30 to 40 grams of carbs (consisting of up to 10 grams of fiber and up to 2 to 3 grams of sugar), up to 5 grams of fat, zero to 50 grams of sodium, and zero grams of cholesterol.

Healthy Food Label

The nutrition facts label for a healthy food should be low in fat, sodium, and sugar. In this example, notice the low sodium, sugar, saturated fat and cholesterol and the high protein and fiber with a few grams of healthy fats.

Healthy Nutrition Facts Label

Serving size	1/2 cup
Servings per container	4
Calories	200
Total fat	2g
Saturated fat	0g
Monounsaturated fat	1g
Polyunsaturated fat	1g
Cholesterol	0mg
Sodium	0mg
Total carbs	20g
Dietary fiber	8g
Sugars	0g
Protein	26g

Unhealthy foods are obvious from their labels. They are high in calories for the serving size and contain large amounts of sodium, cholesterol, sugars and saturated fat. They're also low in protein, monounsaturated fat, polyunsaturated fat, and fiber.

Unhealthy Nutrition Facts Label

Serving size	1/2 cup
Servings per container	4
Calories	200
Total fat	9g
Saturated fat	8g
Monounsaturated fat	0g
Polyunsaturated fat	0g
Trans fat	1g
Cholesterol	200mg
Sodium	810mg

Total carbs	26g
Dietary fiber	0g
Sugars	16g
Protein	4g

My Approach to the Food Label

I use the nutrition facts label selectively. If I am buying whole foods such as meat, potatoes, vegetables, or salad, I really don't need a food label. But if I am buying a processed, prepared food product, then I read the food label very carefully. Cereal is a perfect example. Whenever I am shopping for cereal, I always spend some time to really examine all the different cereals that claim to be healthy. Catchy words such as "sugar-free" and "high-fiber" definitely draw my attention. However, when I look more carefully at these products, more often than not I am surprised by how misleading the label is. Often a so-called "high-fiber" cereal is loaded with high-fructose corn syrup and sodium. It might be high in fiber, but it's also loaded with sugar. I may spend some time examining food labels but eventually I always find the healthiest cereal available. That's almost always a whole-grain cereal with no sugar added.

All-natural whole foods, such as eggs, milk, vegetables, fruit, nuts, fish, seafood, and meat, really don't require strict scrutiny of the food labels. However, foods that are semi-prepared need to be examined for their nutritional contents. These foods would include canned and packaged beans (check their sodium content), cheese, canned vegetables, canned fruit (check for added sugar), protein bars, protein shakes, peanut butter, frozen dinners, and all other types of cake mixes, bread mixes, puddings and potato/stuffing mixes. When buying any of these products, beware of false and catchy claims and carefully examine their nutritional labels. You can still eat all of these foods because, as I have learned, there is always a healthier option. Here are a few examples of how to get good nutrition from packaged foods:

- Pudding and dessert mixes: look for sugar-free, artificially sweetened
- Potato/stuffing mixes: look for high-fiber, sugar, salt-free options
- Frozen dinners: look for low-sodium, low-fat choices
- Bread mixes: look for oat bran, oatmeal options
- Peanut butter: all-natural version
- Protein bars, shakes: sugar-free, high-fiber
- Canned foods: low sodium
- Dehydrated food: low sodium
- Packaged nuts: no salt added
- Popcorn: light version, no salt, no butter added
- Powdered drink mixes: sugar-free, artificially sweetened

When you compare several brands of the same product and look at the labels, it's easy to choose the healthiest brand. You will really be surprised at how the nutritional contents vary from brand to brand. Food marketers are very clever in wording their product's claims to make them seem healthy. Ignore the front of the label where the hype is and carefully read and compare the nutrition facts instead.

15: Proper Meal Planning

As a parent, you should pretty much be able to properly construct perfect meals by now because you now know all of the food categories, why your body needs them, and how to prepare a balanced meal. In this chapter, I will be a little more specific and detailed in order for you to really be able to eat the best meals possible, meals that will bring your body to the next level in appearance and performance. Not only will you learn how to prepare a nutritious meal that will help you become lean and toned, you will also be able to have that same meal be delicious, and without sacrificing any health benefits for flavor.

When most people think of dieting, they think of food that doesn't taste good and that is boring to eat. This is not the case at all! Look for that extra edge when getting into shape. That edge means getting better and easier results, of course. It is all about making the choices that best suit your lifestyle and individual tastes. Keeping it simple is what a long-term commitment is all about. That is how success is achieved: by slow and steady progress that is an enjoyable diet and exercise regimen.

Healthy Meals for Beginners
Standard Menu

Breakfast	2 whole omega-3 eggs
	1 cup high-fiber bran cereal with skim milk
Snack	1 kiwi
Lunch	1 can light tuna with brown rice
Snack	1 fruit

Dinner	lean steak (London broil)
	mashed sweet potatoes made with skim milk
	salad with olive oil, black olives
	sugar-free, fat-free yogurt
Snack	2 tablespoons all-natural peanut butter

Meatless Menu

Breakfast	1 cup artificially sweetened oatmeal mixed with
	1 scoop whey protein isolate
Snack	sugar-free, fat-free yogurt
Lunch	1 hard-boiled omega-3 egg
	2 slices whole-grain bread
Snack	1 fruit
Dinner	steamed clams
	broiled salmon with pepper, lemon, oregano
	watermelon
Snack	8 to 10 almonds

Vegan Menu

Breakfast	high-fiber English muffin with all-natural peanut
	butter and all-natural high-fiber preserves
Snack	1/4 cup walnuts
Lunch	soft tofu with salad, olive oil, vinegar, cashews
Snack	1 fruit
Dinner	extra-firm tofu with fresh tomato sauce and
	whole-grain pasta
	fresh fruit cup
Sanck	2 tablespoons all-natural peanut butter

Healthy Meals for Intermediates

Standard Menu

Breakfast	1/2 cup egg whites cooked with olive oil spray
	1/2 cup all-natural oat bran with artificial sweetener
	1 fruit
Snack	sugar-free, fat-free yogurt
Lunch	grilled chicken breast on whole-wheat bread, mustard
	cucumber and onion salad
Snack	1 fruit
Dinner	broiled eye-round steak
	sautéed spinach
	steamed corn with all-natural butter
	sugar-free pudding
Snack	8 to 10 almonds

Meatless Menu

Breakfast	1 scoop whey protein with 1 cup low-fat cottage cheese
Snack	rice cakes with all-natural peanut butter and
	all-natural jelly
Lunch	canned salmon with wild rice
Snack	1 fruit
Dinner	steamed shrimp and lobster
	1 cup Kashi
	green salad
	sugar-free, fat-free rice pudding
Snack	8 walnuts

Vegan Menu

Breakfast	1 scoop soy protein isolate blended with nuts and oats
Snack	1 fruit
Lunch	brown rice with lentils and onion sautéed with olive oil
Snack	2 tablespoons all-natural peanut butter

Dinner	corn tortillas with beans
	salad with walnuts, olive oil and greens
	whole-wheat pasta with olive oil
	fruit cup
Snack	8 to 10 almonds

16: Portion Size and Control

In addition to eating too much fat and sugar, we often consume an excessive amount of calories because we eat large portions, especially of carbohydrate (starchy) foods. In this chapter, you'll learn how to limit calories by controlling the portion size, using the different food groups as a guide.

As your child's activity level increases as weight loss is achieved, his caloric intake may be increased. Whether or not your kid needs to lose weight, children need to eat a only the number of calories they need to stay healthy and fuel their growth, but not more than what is good for them. Discuss your child's weight and ideal calorie intake with your pediatrician. Use the chart below as a general guide to daily calories for kids who need to lose weight.

Calorie Intake for Weight Loss

Age	Average Daily Calories Needed	Calories for Weight Loss
7–10 (male and female)	1,600–2,200	1,200–1,600
11–14 (male)	2,200–2,800	1,500–2,000
11–14 (female)	1,600–2,400	1,200–1,800
15–18 (male)	2,400–3,400	1,800–2,400
15–18 (female)	1,800–2,400	1,200–1,800

Calories, of course, are very important to monitor. Equally important is portion control and meal frequency. Knowing when to eat foods, and how much of each food group to eat, is extremely critical. For example, if you are burning 3,000 calories per day (later I will teach you all about the amount of calories that your body burns), you must either eat the same amount of calories if you want to maintain your weight, or eat 500 less calories per day if you want to lose a pound of body fat per week. Finally, you would need to eat 300 calories extra per day in order to properly gain weight. Later I will be very specific about calorie and meal breakdowns because, as your nutritional and fitness level increases, so must your attention focus upon how many calories you are to eat and at which times of the day.

Controlling your portions is a necessary step. Eating until you are full is the wrong approach, even when the foods you eat are high-protein, quality foods. Eating without measuring your portion size will expand your stomach gradually, which means that you will need more and more food to feel satisfied. You must control your portions to a point where you are eating four to six small meals each day and each meal consists of fiber, water, 25 to 45 grams of protein, 25 to 50 grams of carbohydrates, and less than 9 grams of healthy fat.

All vegetables, with the exception of tomatoes and corn, can be eaten without restriction. Eating plenty of vegetables gives you a feeling of fullness without unwanted calories, plus vegetables have a lot of other health benefits. By adding plenty of vegetables to your diet, you will have a much easier time staying lean or getting into shape. For me, eating vegetables is a great way to stay lean and fit but without suffering and feeling hungry all of the time. A lot of my success in dieting and staying lean I owe to eating vegetables. You can never eat too many of them!

Eating the proper foods in the right quantities is really the secret to success for achieving your fitness goals. To be sure you're getting the proper portions of the right foods, measure them with tools such as measuring cups, digital scales, and tablespoons. Use the chart below to get an idea of how proper food portions are measured.

Proteins	*Precooked Portion Size*
Meat and poultry	5–7 ounces
Egg whites	4–7 egg whites or 2/3 cup liquid egg whites
Whey or soy protein isolate	2 ounces
Fish	6 ounces
nonfat Greek yogurt	1 cup
nonfat cottage cheese	1 cup
Tofu (firm)	5–7 ounces
Seafood	8–10 ounces
Canned/pouched seafood	5–7 ounces
Skim milk	20 ounces

Carbohydrates	*Portion Size*
Sweet potato	4–8 ounces
Rice (brown or wild)	1/2–3/4 cup
Pasta (whole-wheat)	1 cup
Old-fashioned oats	1/2–3/4 cup
Oat bran	1/3–1/2 cup
Unprocessed wheat bran	1/2–2/3 cup
Sugar-free bran cereal	1 cup
Quinoa	2/3 cup
Kashi	1 cup
Bagel (whole-grain)	1/2 bagel
Bread (whole-grain)	2 slices
Rice cakes (plain)	3 pieces
High-fiber waffles	2 pieces
Beans	2/3 cup
Lentils	1 cup
Vegetable soup	1 cup
Cream of wheat	1/2 cup
Cream of rice	1/2 cup

Sugar-free, nonfat pudding	2/3 cup
Nonfat cheese	3/4 cup
High-fiber breakfast muffin	1 piece
Sugar-free, nonfat yogurt	3/4 cup
Sugar-free, nonfat ice cream	3/4 cup
Italian ice (sugar-free)	1 cup

Fruit	*Portion Size*
Apple	4–6 ounces
Banana	1 small
Pear	4–6 ounces
Grapes	1 cup
Blueberries	1 cup
Raspberries	1 cup
Blackberries	1 cup
Kiwi	4–6 ounces
Peach	4–6 ounces
Orange	1 small
Grapefruit	1/2 grapefruit

Note: All other fruit portions should be either 1 cup or 4–6 ounces, which would be the equivalent of 1 small piece of fruit.

Fats	*Portion Size*
Extra virgin olive oil	1 tablespoon
Canola oil	1 tablespoon
Avocado	4 ounces
Coconut	3 ounces
Peanut butter	2 tablespoons
Nuts	1/4 cup
Butter	1 teaspoon
Eggs	1 per day
Flaxseeds	1/4 cup

| Flaxseed oil | 1 tablespoon |

Vegetables	*Portion Size*
Tomato	up to 3 small pieces
Corn	3/4 cup kernels or 1 whole cob

Note: Eat as much as you want of all other vegetables.

17: Customized Healthy Meals

We are now going to the next level of meal planning. I call this "meal customization" because, with this method, the meals are constructed in a way that best suits your taste, fitness goals, and daily routine, which depends upon how active you really are. Whether you are a child, teenager or parent, it doesn't matter: there is always a specific diet that will work best for you. In this chapter you will learn the difference between diets that are used to gain muscle mass, gain strength, lose weight, increase endurance, and most importantly, improve the quality of your life.

There is no question that this isn't an overnight process but one that, if followed properly, will render results that no amount of money could ever buy! Notice that as you continue reading the meal plans become more and more specific. That enables you to use the meal plan that best suits your fitness goals and tastes. Each and every diet has its specific purpose. Before beginning any type of meal plan, you must first know what is it that you are looking to achieve from it. Remember that there are many ways to get to the same destination.

Meals for the Overweight and Inactive Child

An overweight and inactive child would initially seem like the most difficult to work with and see any type of success with weight loss. This is not true at all because, when it comes to losing weight, it is all just simple mathematics: the number of calories that are eaten must be less than the number of calories that the body burns throughout the day. The chart below has meal plan suggestions that will help an inactive child lose weight.

Beginning Meal Plans for Overweight and Inactive Children

Note: Avoid sugary sodas, juice, and other soft drinks. Choose artificially sweetened beverages, but remember that plain water is the best choice. Aim for 2 to 4 quarts a day, depending on the age of the child.

Standard Menu #1

Breakfast	1 cup high-fiber, sugar-free bran cereal
	1 hard-boiled omega-3 egg
Snack	1 fruit
Lunch	5 oz. grilled chicken breast
	green salad
Snack	1 fruit
Dinner	5 oz. eye round steak
	steamed vegetables with nonfat seasoning
	or dressing
Snack	1 fruit

Meatless Menu #1

Breakfast	1/2 cup old-fashioned oats with blueberries
	and 1 scoop whey protein
Snack	1 fruit
Lunch	grilled fish with no-salt seasoning
	cucumber and onion salad
Snack	1 fruit
Dinner	fish baked with garlic and lemon
	salad with olive oil, vinegar, onions, peppers,
	lettuce
Snack	1 fruit

Vegan Menu #1

Breakfast	1 glass nonfat rice milk
	1/2 whole-grain bagel with all-natural fruit
	preserves

Snack	1 fruit
Lunch	salad with greens, flaxseeds, olive oil, vinegar and walnuts
	1 cup wild rice mixed with lentils
	1 small fruit
Snack	8 to 10 almonds
Dinner	extra-firm tofu sautéed with onion, shallots and garlic
	steamed red beans mixed with corn
Snack	1 fruit

Standard Menu #2

Breakfast	nonfat cheese
	1 cup strawberries with nonfat whipped cream
Snack	1 fruit
Lunch	lean ground beef mixed with corn and Brussels sprouts
	1/2 cantaloupe
Snack	2 tablespoons all-natural peanut butter
Dinner	5 oz. grilled turkey breast
	baked vegetable combination (cauliflower, onion, butternut squash sprinkled with a little extra virgin olive oil)
	sugar-free jello
Snack	1 fruit

Meatless Menu

Breakfast	1/2 cup egg whites cooked with olive oil spray
	1 banana
Snack	10 walnuts

Lunch	1 can tuna in olive oil mixed with peas and vinegar
Snack	1 fruit
Dinner	5 oz. broiled fish with no-salt seasoning baked butternut squash with melted nonfat cheese 1 cup sugar-free, nonfat pudding
Snack	1 fruit

Vegan Menu

Breakfast	2/3 cup old-fashioned oatmeal mixed with 1 scoop soy protein isolate and 8 almonds
Lunch	1 cup cooked black beans with whole-grain pasta and all-natural tomato sauce
Snack	1 fruit
Dinner	baked tofu with tomatoes, olive oil and onion BBQ corn on the cob sugar-free Italian ice
Snack	1 fruit

On any weight-loss diet, the primary goal is to avoid starchy carbohydrate such as potatoes, rice, and pasta. Instead of these starchy carbohydrates, fill up with plenty of vegetables and fruits. Overall, aim for more veggies than fruit. Keep fruit portions small. The best and most effective times to eat fruit are with breakfast and immediately following a workout.

The beginner's diet for the inactive, overweight child will help give you an understanding of how to help your child eat in a way that will lead to weight loss without hunger while teaching the child what a healthy diet should be. After a while, however, your child may need to move on to the intermediate version. This will be necessary if weight loss has slowed before the child reaches the desired weight. Whenever you diet, your body eventually adjusts and progress slows down. The intermediate version should jump start your body into its fat-burning mode again.

Meal Plans for Overweight and Inactive Children

Note: Avoid sugary sodas, juice, and other soft drinks. Choose artificially sweetened beverages, but remember that plain water is the best choice. Aim for 2 to 4 quarts a day, depending on the age of the child.

Standard Menu

Breakfast	1/2 cup scrambled egg whites with nonfat cheese
	high-fiber English muffin
Snack	carrot and celery sticks with low-fat cream cheese
Lunch	tuna wrap made with light tuna in water, nonfat mayonnaise, lettuce, onion, on a high-fiber, low-carb wrap
Dinner	6 oz. grilled chicken breast with mushrooms and olive oil
	red beet salad with olive oil and vinegar
	1 fruit

Meatless Menu

Breakfast	2 pancakes made with egg whites, oatmeal, skim milk and honey, served with sugar-free syrup
Snack	protein pudding made with whey protein, water, ice, cinnamon and refrigerated
Lunch	6 oz. cooked lean chopped meat mixed with corn, onion, and low-fat cheddar cheese
Dinner	grilled seafood in lemon and garlic

Greek salad (nonfat feta cheese, black olives, lettuce, onion, tomato, black pepper, olive oil, vinegar and lemon)

sugar-free, nonfat gelato with walnuts on top

Vegan Menu

Breakfast	soy protein pudding made with 2 oz. soy protein isolate, water, ice, blueberries, blended and refrigerated
Snack	1 cup strawberries blended with 1 cup skim milk
Lunch	sautéed broccoli rabe with garlic, lentils, and corn, olive oil
Dinner	tofu baked with mushrooms, red pepper, onion and tomato sauce chopped strawberry, blackberry and kiwi blended with nonfat soy milk, refrigerated and served as pudding
Snack	8 to 10 almonds

The intermediate meal plan provides more calories. This is because the more frequently you eat, the more your metabolism increases; hence, so does your body's need for calories. So, on this plan, you eat more food and eat more frequently. Amazingly, your body will still burn more fat! This process must be carefully monitored with the proper food and calories and what time of day meals are eaten. Consistency is what it's all about!

Once your child has achieved the desired weight loss, he or she has reached the advanced level. This level includes eating more frequently, and more calories, thus making it easy to maintain the weight loss.

Advanced Meal Plans for the Overweight and Inactive Child

Note: Avoid sugary sodas, juice, and other soft drinks. Choose artificially sweetened beverages, but remember that plain water is the best choice. Aim for 2 to 4 quarts a day, depending on the age of the child.

Standard Menu

Breakfast	2/3 cup unprocessed wheat bran
	8 almonds
	1 cup nonfat Greek yogurt
Snack	1 fruit
Lunch	1 high-fiber, low-carb wrap with lettuce and
	1 can salmon mixed with mustard
	1 fruit
Snack	1 pickle
Dinner	6 oz. lean pork broiled with lemon and olive oil
	collard greens with nonfat sour cream
	sugar-free, nonfat yogurt with walnuts

Meatless Menu

Breakfast	2/3 cup of egg whites and 1 yolk scrambled with nonfat sharp cheese
Snack	1 glass nonfat soy milk
Lunch	1 cup mixed corn kernels and carrots slices with 4 oz. chicken breast seasoned with vinegar and pepper
Snack	1 scoop whey protein isolate mixed with 1 glass of water
Dinner	1 lb. steamed lobster
	sautéed cauliflower with olive oil
	garden salad with vinegar and olive oil
	frozen sugar-free fruit bar

Vegan Menu

Breakfast	8 oz. nonfat rice milk blended with 1 cup nonfat soy milk, 1 cup strawberries, ice and water
Snack	1 fruit
Lunch	lentil soup
	1 low-fat, low-carb, high-fiber tortilla
Snack	1 cup strawberries
Dinner	green beans, beets, garlic, broccoli, low-fat tofu, crushed red pepper

In the advanced diet, your child is now eating more food and more frequently because his or her metabolism has naturally increased due to the calorie restriction and meal frequency. As you increase the amount of calories, it increases the need for more calories for the body to sustain itself. With this now faster metabolism your body is more alert, energized, and more efficiently burning its own body fat! Yes, it is a science and may seem too good to be true, but you will witness it for yourself. You'll be eating more food and losing weight, all at the same time!

Meals for the Overweight and Active Child

There are many active children out there who are also overweight. At first this surprised me, because these kids are burning a lot of calories every day. How could they be overweight? The answer is that they were simply consuming too many calories, because in our society food is everywhere. They were eating too many unhealthy snacks, both at school and in their after-school programs. Even when their parents were careful to serve healthy meals at home, their kids were getting unhealthy food elsewhere.

Working with active overweight kids is an easier task because they already have the drive and competitiveness to participate in sports and exercise. They need more calories in their diets because of the extra calories they burn throughout the day. The diet plans below are designed to reduce calories but give these kids the extra complex carbohydrates they need to fuel their activity.

Beginning Meal Plans for the Overweight and Active Child

Note: Avoid sugary sodas, juice, and other soft drinks. Choose artificially sweetened beverages, but remember that plain water is the best choice. Aim for 2 to 4 quarts a day, depending on the age of the child.

Standard Menu

Breakfast	2 high-fiber pancakes with sugar-free syrup
	2 hard-boiled omega-3 eggs
	1 cup orange juice
Snack	1 fruit
Lunch	1.5 oz. grilled turkey breast with high-fiber English muffin
Snack	1 fruit
Dinner	grilled London broil
	1/2 cup wild rice
	garden salad with olive oil and vinegar
	nonfat, sugar-free pudding
Snack	1 fruit

Meatless Menu

Breakfast	1/2 cup scrambled egg whites
	1 high-fiber English muffin with high-fiber preserves
Snack	1 fruit
Lunch	5 oz. grilled salmon
	cucumber salad
Snack	1 fruit
Dinner	steamed clams, scallops with lemon and olive oil

	1/2 cup whole grain pasta, olive oil
	steamed broccoli
	1 fruit

Vegan Menu

Breakfast	2 slices rye toast with all-natural preserves
	1 cup nonfat Greek yogurt with 8 almonds, rice milk
Snack	1 fruit
Lunch	1 high-fiber, low-carb pita with 2 tablespoons all-natural peanut butter
	1 fruit
Snack	1 fruit
Dinner	1 cup brown rice mixed with 3/4 cup pinto beans
	green salad with olive oil and vinegar
	sugar-free Italian ice
Snack	1 fruit

The beginner's meal plan for the overweight active child includes a few more complex carbohydrates in order to provide needed extra calories and energy. The beginner should only need to eat three times per day because that is a good starting point to eventually increasing the amount of meals per day in order to speed up the body's metabolism.

The beginner's meal plan starts really right at the supermarket, where the healthy foods are purchased. The junk food is no longer bought nor kept anywhere in the house. A child's snacks of cookies and cakes are now, instead, fruits and nuts; sodas are now sugar-free drinks or plain water.

Are you understanding the mechanics behind the psychology of eating and living right? This is what I call the lifestyle for attaining a good quality of life. So many people think that "quality of life" means material things, like having a lot of money, a nice home, and a fancy car. But if you are overweight and miserable inside, and hiding behind the expensive home and car, is your life a good one? In reality, quality of life means happiness. So how happy can you be if you are fifty pounds overweight, have a puffy red face, and are too embarrassed to wear shorts? Or being the child that is never picked to play on a team or who is laughed at by the other kids? To me, that sounds like a sad situation for anyone. The good news is that it is easily correctable! A simple meal plan and exercise routine is all that you need in order to find a better way of life. So why not make a few small sacrifices that will yield tremendous and life changing dividends?

When I was a child, I was extremely hungry for dietary information but had no clue where to start. At fourteen, I received the fantastic gift of a weight set and began lifting weights immediately. At the same time, I was a freshman on the high school wrestling team and was learning how to lose weight. All I needed to lose was a mere seven pounds, because I was tired of losing to other wrestlers who were bigger and stronger than me. If I lost the seven pounds, I could compete at a lower weight class and have greater success. That's what I did—and that's when it all began for me. The lifestyle of exercise and proper nutrition became a part of my life at fourteen and still is today. It has been a wonderful ride and it's still going on!

Intermediate Meal Plans for the Overweight and Active Child

Note: Avoid sugary sodas, juice, and other soft drinks. Choose artificially sweetened beverages, but remember that plain water is the best choice. Aim for 2 to 4 quarts a day, depending on the age of the child.

Standard Menu

Breakfast	2 oatmeal and honey pancakes with sugar-free syrup
	1 cup skim milk
	1 cup all-natural juice
Lunch	1 cup whole-wheat pasta with nonfat cheddar cheese, black pepper mixed with

	3 oz. chicken breast
Snack	1 can light all-natural pineapple
Dinner	meatloaf made with 90% lean ground beef
	cauliflower topped with 1 tablespoon butter
	fruit smoothie (blended watermelon,
	cantaloupe and blueberries)

Meatless Menu

Breakfast	scrambled egg whites with salsa and
	low-fat cheese
	1/2 whole-wheat bagel
	1 banana
Lunch	grilled shrimp with garlic, olive oil and lem
	on mixed with zucchini, corn and chopped
	carrots
	1 cup blueberries with nonfat whipped cream
Snack	celery and carrot sticks with fat-free dip
Dinner	broiled fish with lentils, onion and red pepper
	sweet potato with nonfat sour cream and
	cheddar cheese
	sliced banana and kiwi with nonfat
	whipped cream

Vegan Menu

Breakfast	1/2 cup oatmeal mixed with 2 tablespoons
	all-natural peanut butter
	1 cup nonfat soy milk
Snack	1 small pear
Lunch	baked vegetable mix with cauliflower,
	broccoli, Brussels sprouts, olive oil
	1 whole-wheat pita bread
	8 almonds

Snack	1 glass nonfat rice milk
Dinner	baked tofu with chopped vegetables
	baked sweet potato
	1 sugar-free frozen fruit bar

The intermediate diet contains more calories and one snack. As you gradually move up the ladder and eventually reach the advanced meal plan, you will begin to feel more hungry and energized. This means that your body's metabolism is slowly but surely increasing. When this positive change occurs, it is important to slowly increase your calories to enable your body burn the increased amount of calories without converting them to fat. During this process your body slowly adjusts itself to where it is needing more and more calories in order to sustain itself. At this point, you will be able to eat more food and lose body fat at the same time. This is our goal, to turn your body into a fat-burning and high-revving machine! Follow the formula that I am organizing for you and this will happen. You will love the results!

Meal Proportions

For the overweight and inactive child, prepare meals based on the following proportions:

• Protein: 20 to 25 grams per meal
• Fat: less than 9 grams per meal, preferably mono- and polyunsaturated fats
• Carbohydrates: less than 30 grams
• Fiber: as much as possible from vegetables, salad, and fruit

For the overweight but active child, the meal proportions are similar except for the addition of a few more grams of simple carbs following exercise, and a few more complex carbs throughout the day. Remember that it is very important for the inactive, overweight child to eat vegetables as their carbohydrates. Vegetables and protein together make an excellent meal to lose body fat and body weight at a quick pace. This has been my secret for years, whenever I needed to lose extra body fat in a rather short time. Eat plenty of vegetables to reduce your hunger and maintain great health in your digestive tract.

You have a lot of meal choices. I want you to choose the ones that will make your weight loss transition as easy and as fun as possible. I always tell people, this is a marathon and not a sprint. Improving your health and body will take a while to accomplish, so choose a comfortable pace that you can sustain.

Meals for the Underweight and Inactive Child

Many children are underweight. These kids come home from school and head right for the computer or video games for hours on end. Often they go without eating until dinner. These children become very weak as well as thin because of a lack of physical exertion and because they are indoors for most of the day. Aside from the damage to their growth and long-term health, these kids can lose their self-esteem and confidence. This is a direction we never want to see anyone head toward because it causes so much pain and suffering.

Beginner Meal Plans for the Underweight and Inactive Child

Note: Avoid sugary sodas, juice, and other soft drinks. Choose artificially sweetened beverages, but remember that plain water is the best choice. Aim for 2 to 4 quarts a day, depending on the age of the child.

Standard Menu

Breakfast	2 whole omega-3 eggs with cheese
	2 slices whole wheat toast with butter and high-fiber all-natural preserves
Lunch	93% lean beef hamburger with cheese on whole-grain bun
	1 low-fat yogurt with fruit and nonfat whipped cream
Dinner	1/2 baked chicken with no-salt seasoning sweet potato with butter

broccoli with melted cheese
1 scoop low-fat sugar-free ice cream
with walnuts

Meatless Menu

Breakfast 2 whole-grain waffles with all-natural
peanut butte
scrambled egg whites with 1 yolk
1 cup 100% fruit juice

Lunch grilled low-fat cheese sandwich on rye bread
1 banana

Dinner broiled salmon with capers and lemon with
olive oil
1 cup brown rice with peas
Greek salad
sugar-free Italian ice

Vegan Menu

Breakfast 1/2 cup walnuts
1 cup 100% fruit juice
1 cup low-fat rice milk
1/2 cup oatmeal with all-natural
peanut butter

Lunch 1 cup wild rice with black beans
garden salad
1 fruit

Dinner tomatoes with tofu and onion
sweet potato
sautéed broccoli rabe with olive oil and garlic
frozen pudding made with nonfat soy milk

Intermediate Meal Plans for the Underweight and Inactive Child

Note: Avoid sugary sodas, juice, and other soft drinks. Choose artificially sweetened beverages, but remember that plain water is the best choice. Aim for two to four quarts a day, depending on the age of the child.

Standard Menu

Breakfast	low-fat Greek yogurt with fruit
	high-fiber English muffin with butter and
	high-fiber natural preserves
	1 cup 100% orange juice
Lunch	4 oz. chicken breast stir-fried with vegetables,
	served in a low-carb high-fiber wrap
	1/2 cup blackberries
Snack	1 small bag dried fruit and nuts
	(sugar- and salt-free)
Dinner	5 oz. lean pork chop
	1 cup lentil soup with whole-grain pasta
	1 cup corn and spinach with butter
	1 slice low-fat, sugar-free cheesecake

Meatless Menu

Breakfast	2 oatmeal and honey high-fiber pancakes
	with sugar-free syrup and fat-free
	whipped cream
	8 oz. orange juice
Lunch	3 oz. salmon mixed with onion, light
	mayonnaise, shredded low-fat cheese in
	a high-fiber multigrain wrap
Snack	1 slice watermelon
Dinner	eggplant parmigiana made with low-fat
	mozzarella

sautéed onions and mushrooms with olive oil
and crushed red pepper
1 slice sugar-free apple pie with a scoop of
low-fat sugar-free yogurt

Vegan Menu

Breakfast	1/2 cup quinoa or oat bran with 8 walnuts
	1 cup low-fat soy milk
	1 low-fat muffin
Lunch	2/3 cup of refried beans with low-fat,
	high-fiber corn tortilla
	sugar-free fruit cocktail
Snack	2 tablespoons all-natural peanut butter
Dinner	1 cup wild rice mixed with red beans
	and corn
	hearts of palm and black olive salad
	fruit cup

The intermediate plan allows you to eat more calories than the beginner plan. With the added calories, this plan will slowly help speed up your metabolism so that your body burns more fat and builds muscle at the same time. By eating small meals, your body gets a steady intake of high-quality calories. Eating these meals will also provide you with so much more energy throughout the day. More energy equals more fun, more activities, and more accomplishments.

The intermediate diet for the inactive underweight individual consists of plenty of fruit and higher fat proteins. This individual will feel more energized and his body will feel tighter. Eating in this manner will provide the leaner individual with plenty of protein and nutrients that will feed the muscle and make it grow and become stronger; hence the child's appetite will increase. A child with a good appetite means that he or she is healthy and eating properly because leaner and protein-rich foods burn a lot faster in the body, making the child hungry more often. Eating frequently will give your body an enormous amount of energy. This will help the inactive child want to become more active. Eating properly can drastically change your lifestyle for the better!

Advanced Meal Plans for the Underweight and Inactive Child

Note: Avoid sugary sodas, juice, and other soft drinks. Choose artificially sweetened beverages, but remember that plain water is the best choice. Aim for two to four quarts a day, depending on the age of the child.

Standard Menu

Breakfast	2 whole omega-3 eggs with low-fat sour cream and spinach
	1 low-fat bran muffin
	8 walnuts
Snack	1 low-sugar, low-fat energy bar
Lunch	5 oz. grilled chicken on whole-grain bread with low-fat sharp cheese, onion, tomato, lettuce
	1 fruit
Snack	1 cup sugar- and salt-free trail mix
Dinner	5 oz. London broil with sautéed mushrooms, onions, red pepper, garlic and olive oil
	Greek salad
	sweet potato with butter
	rice pudding made with brown rice, Splenda, skim milk, cinnamon

Meatless Menu

Breakfast	low-fat cheese blintzes
	2/3 cup scrambled egg whites with green pepper and mushroom

	1 cup 100% fruit juice
Snack	1 glass low-fat chocolate milk
Lunch	1 can light tuna with low-fat salad dressing and onion, served in a low-fat high-fiber pita
	1 cup of red grapes
Snack	1 small piece melon
Dinner	grilled seafood combination with lemon and olive oil
	1 cup whole-wheat pasta with low-fat grated cheese and olive oil
	cucumber and tomato salad
	smoothie made with blended walnuts, skim milk, blueberries, ice and water, blended together

Vegan Menu

Breakfast	protein shake with 1 scoop of soy protein isolate, 5 almonds, 1/2 cup old-fashioned oats, 1/2 cup white grapes, ice and water
Snack	1 glass low-fat rice milk
Lunch	1 cup brown rice mixed with navy beans
	garden salad with olives
	1 small can sugar-free fruit cocktail
Snack	1 fruit
Dinner	vegetable casserole with low-fat extra-firm tofu and lentils
	fresh fruit cup with almond or soy milk

The advanced version will provide your body with the necessary nutrition to fuel and strengthen the muscles. Once a child begins to eat in this format, by the time he becomes a teenager, he will be able to eat more calories and not become overweight, and he will most likely be much stronger than most if not all of his peers. The child who becomes aware of his diet at such a young age will be at such an advantage later on by having better health and quality of life. Eating healthy will also increase the child's confidence and athletic ability, along with overall feeling of happiness.

18: Fitness for Children and Pre-Teens

I am a firm believer that exercise benefits everyone, including those with mental illnesses such as depression, anxiety, and low self-esteem. After anyone exercises, they experience an unbelievably euphoric feeling. After exercising you feel as if you no longer have a problem in the world! It's a fantastic feeling! When a child is in a sad or tired mood, have him or her exercise or do something active, and within thirty minutes he or she will feel a lot better!

When children are at this age, their personalities are beginning to develop. It's crucial for them to mentally develop in a healthy way—and there is no healthier way than developing confidence. Once a child feels confident, he or she feels that they have worth and can accomplish anything.

You may be thinking that this all sounds great, but how can you get your child to exercise? Through motivation and education. Education, meaning applying all of the nutritional and exercise programs into your child's lifestyle; and motivation, meaning to relate these programs to your child in a way that makes him or her really want to do this as opposed to feeling obligated to follow the program.

A good motivating technique is to lead by example. You can do this by preparing healthy meals for the entire family so that everyone eats the same food. The same applies to exercising: you should follow the programs together and engage in the same sports where possible as well (bike riding, for example), because your child will look up to you for spending quality time together. Remember, parents: don't be lazy!

Athletic Fitness Program

An athletic fitness program is a fun, creative approach to improving athletic abilities. It is important to break down the program into five components. They are: coordination, stamina, strength, speed, and agility. The program will help the child improve in each category, which will help the child perform much better, not just in sports but in all activities of daily living. By developing in these areas of fitness, the training will become easier as time passes and you will be very motivated because you will see improvements as you go along.

Exercising can range from simple and basic all the way to sports specific. By implementing this system, you will quickly notice improvement both on and off the playing field. Your kids will even walk and talk with more confidence. The fact is many athletes don't reach their true natural athletic potential and never achieve their ultimate peak performance because they didn't learn the basics when they were young. Long gone are the days when nearly every child experienced physical activity every day they attended school. Today, students are lucky to get an hour a week of any type of organized physical activity and fitness. Many kids don't even want to go out and play anymore. Unfortunately, creativity, fitness, and athletic skills are no longer developed in the backyard, schoolyard, or parks.

During sports practice, time must be spent on developing overall movement skills. Doing so will make coaching more effective and rewarding, and each child's athletic experience will be more enjoyable and beneficial. Skateboarders, snowboarders, and BMX riders have the right idea. These athletes focus on free play with friends and on developing their creativity and athletic and fitness skills. They spend hours, days, and years on perfecting tricks by experimenting with combinations of athletic movements. For many years, the sports community look down on these athletes because of their different attitudes about traditional sports. Surprisingly, these kids are now some of the most physically fit and well-trained athletes among the new generation. In their creative tricks and maneuvers they are developing all of the athletic components: coordination, stamina, strength, speed, and agility.

With fundamentally sound training, your child will not develop bad habits—this is extremely important. When bad habits, such as poor running form, are created they become very difficult to correct. Another concern in kids' sports is that many kids choose to participate in only one sport in order to master it and participate in it all year. This means no real rest and recovery for body parts continually used over an extended period of time. Combine this with the execution of the same drills over the course of a season, or over an entire year, and you have many young athletes running a high risk for overuse injuries. The correct training method includes variations of drills and many options for improving all areas of fitness. The goal is to balance activities and competitions to better develop and prepare the athlete's future performance, health, and fitness. By constantly changing the training routines, you take repeated stress off any one body part, thus avoiding overuse injuries. Training doesn't have to be boring and it doesn't have to feel like work. Sports and athletic development doesn't need to be taught the same way it is been taught for years. Most importantly, whenever exercising, whether it's in the backyard, gym, or field, develop your full potential. It's all about having fun and being in shape. And winning is fun too, so definitely make the most of it.

19: Improving Flexibility and Range of Motion

For improving flexibility and range of motion (the distance and direction a joint can move to its full potential), I recommend a series of exercises done before training sessions.

Arm Spins
Stand straight up with your arms fully extended. Circle them in a forward-and-reverse motion and also touch your hands together, putting them directly in front of you. Move your arms from the front to the sides or as far back as you can. Perform for 1 straight minute.

Hip Stretch
Stand straight up while using one arm to support yourself against a wall. Lift your right leg directly in front of you as high as you can. Raise your right leg as high up to the sides and to the rear as you can. Then switch legs and repeat. Perform for 2 straight minutes.

Neck Stretches
Use each of your arms to pull your head from one side to the next. Perform for 1 minute.

Back Stretch
Sit on the floor with your legs straight out in front of you. Extend your arms and reach as forward as you can, trying to touch your toes. Perform for 3 minutes.

Arm and Shoulder Stretch

Reach up and stretch your arms as high as possible while holding your hands. Hold for 30 seconds.

Groin Stretch

Sit on the floor and extend your legs out as far apart from each other as you can. Extend both arms together and try to touch one foot; hold the stretch for 20 seconds. Then repeat with the other leg. Perform for 2 straight minutes.

If you're not sure about how to do these exercises, work with a trainer or coach, or look for videos online.

20: Developing Agility

Agility is the ability to change direction rapidly without losing speed or balance. Agility is important in all activities because it helps you perform better and avoid injury. For improving agility, I recommend the series of exercises listed below three times a week.

Staggered Lunges
Do walking lunges in a zigzag, staggered motion. Perform two 20-yard lunges.

Skip Steps
Skip on each leg for 20 yards each leg.

Basketball Bounce
Dribble a basketball for 20 yards while walking; do 20 yards for each hand. Repeat while running.

Soccer Ball Drill
Kick a soccer ball in short bursts, keeping it close to you, for 20 yards while walking. Repeat while jogging. Next, stand in place and juggle the soccer ball on each leg. Perform two sets of 10 repetitions.

Obstacle Course Run
Place six to eight traffic cones or any other visible object on the ground about five yards apart. Run in a zigzag, figure-eight pattern around all the obstacles. Do 10 repetions for two sets.

Hamstring Stretch

Run up several flights of stairs, skipping every other step. Alternatively, run for 20 yards on a flat surface, taking huge steps—at least three feet per step. Perform for 30 seconds to one minute.

To learn how the exercises should be done, work with a trainer or coach, or look for videos online.

21: Developing Balance

Balance is a necessary requirement in every motion and sport that you do. Balance and coordination work together. Developing balance occurs through constant repetition and a few simple exercises. Balance will help you execute every movement in a way that is graceful and fluid. However, some people seem to be naturally better balanced than others. Balance develops an overall sense of equilibrium, self-control and total body awareness. I consider balance to be the foundation to athletic development. The more balance becomes the focus of a child's athletic development, the more adept he or she will become at performing more difficult and complicated tasks. I will list a few drills and activities that will improve the child's balance and how to control the body in many athletic situations. Whether the exercise is mobile or stationary, single or with a partner, all of these drills will improve balance.

• Two-by-four walk. Place a piece of two-by-four on the ground and walk along it. Walk across five times with one footstep in front of the other, sideways, and zigzag.

• Knee balancing. Kneel on a skateboard and rock back and forth and from side to side. Perform for 1 minute.

• Standing balance. Stand on a skateboard, rocking side to side and back and forth. Perform for 2 minutes.

• Bicycle balance. With both feet on one side of a bike, balance on the pedal for 1 minute. Change sides and repeat for 1 minute.

• Basketball balancing. Bounce a basketball while standing on a skateboard. Perform for 1 minute while dribbling in each hand.

• Tennis drill. Stand on a large pillow while swinging a tennis racket and hitting the ball against a wall. Perform for 2 minutes.

• Two-by-four roll. Walk along a two-by-four and, on the last step, roll forward.

• Basketball push-ups. Put your hands on a basketball and perform 10 push-ups.

• Medicine ball push-ups. Place your toes on a medicine ball and perform 10 push-ups.

• Jumping rope. Jump rope and, with each leg, try to close one eye while jumping. Jump for 5 straight minutes.

To learn how the exercises should be done, work with a trainer or coach, or look for videos online.

22: Increasing Stamina

Stamina is what gets allows the body to keep going over an extended period of time without tiring. Stamina is both physical energy and mental energy. Although it is typically associated with endurance athletes such as marathon runners, every sport, every activity, and every aspect of life requires some level of stamina. Any sport that involves continuous play with no regular rest intervals (such as those that occur between pitches and innings in baseball, for example) needs stamina. Sports such as baseball and softball are slow-paced with little physical exertion, unless you're a pitcher or catcher. Still, baseball is a sport in which stamina must be developed in order to develop strength.

All sports have specific stamina requirements that need to be developed for athletes to perform at optimal levels. Stamina allows athletes to execute the skills of their sport without tiring or losing concentration. When athletes find themselves tiring during a competition, they might become physically unable to execute the skills necessary to excel. For example, a hockey defenseman who tires toward the end of a game might not be able to chase down a puck in his zone, allowing the opposition to gain control and score. Fatigue can also affect concentration and decision-making, such as when a basketball point guard gets tired and misses a pick that was set by a teammate and ends up turning the ball over at a critical point in the game.

Throughout my athletic career, there have been many times when I was too tired to execute the move correctly during a wrestling match. When you are tired, you tend to lose confidence in your ability. If you are in doubt, that leads to hesitation, allowing your opponent to capitalize on the situation. The famous football coach Vince Lombardi said, "Fatigue makes cowards of us all." What this means is that when you are playing sports or doing anything else that is physical, and you become tired, you now want to quit, instead of fighting for that ball, or chasing that hockey puck, or fighting for that takedown during a wrestling match. In other words, when you become tired you don't put that extra "oomph" into the game. Simply put, when you become tired, you give up. In my experience, every time I have given up because of fatigue, for that split second I felt relieved. After a minute or so, once I caught my breath, I felt guilty and like a quitter. Not a good feeling at all!

The good news is that becoming fatigued can be minimized with proper training and exercises. Once you are in good cardiovascular shape, you have a lot more stamina. You feel more confident and able to execute your game strategy and moves in a much more precise manner. When you are tired, you tend to execute your moves and strategy in a sub-par manner. I can't stress to you enough the importance of stamina.

Today's kids spend a lot more time in front of computers, video games, and television sets. They are sedentary for long periods of time at school, including the commute to and from school, with little to no movement other than walking between classes and to lunch. The reduction of physical education has drastically decreased physical activity during school hours. In addition, more schools are finding it difficult to continue after-school activities and sports because of budget constraints. These factors combined have led to a serious decline in overall fitness among a majority of kids and can be quite noticeable when a child plays on an organized sports team. Kid still enjoy running and moving and the freedom that playing provides. But for many, the only chance they have to exercise their stamina is at an organized practice or game. In these settings, endurance does not receive enough attention or is presented in a negative fashion. Unfortunately, stamina training is often applied as a punishment. It should not be presented in a negative way. For example, athletes are sent to run a number of laps or told to do a number of push-ups as a punishment for being late, making a mistake, or misbehaving. This can result in a lifetime of negative feelings toward working out. Because endurance is such an integral part of sports performance, stamina training should never be used as a punishment. It should be presented as a fun activity that promotes positive feelings toward working out. Remember that having fun must be a big part of exercise in order to achieve successful results.

Stamina training should be done strategically. For younger kids, it shouldn't necessarily be conducted separately from the activity or at one particular time during practice. For teens or adults, conditioning exercises should be done separately, depending on the sport. Usually you are improving your conditioning just by playing the actual sport. Splitting up stamina training within a practice should increase the overall intensity each athlete exerts during these segments.

For best results, stamina training should be customized depending on age and level of competition. Stamina training for kids should consist of general activities that are fun and that encourage the athletes to push themselves to their next level of fitness. Many healthy kids of this age have a natural supply of energy that provides them with significant endurance to apply to any sport. But because of the sedentary nature of American society today, stamina training should never be overlooked.

One of the best general methods for building stamina in young kids is to incorporate different sports into their practices. For example, if you coach basketball, take ten minutes during practice to play small side games of soccer or flag football. This allows the kids to perform different movements that they wouldn't normally do in the sport that they normally engaged in. Their overall stamina will improve, because whenever the body is unfamiliar with a particular exercise, the workout seems to improve stamina. Actually, the body will quickly adapt to any workout that is performed frequently, which eventually levels off any increase in stamina. It is always best to shock the body by frequently changing the workouts. By incorporating different sports into conditioning training, you will not only improve the level of stamina but you will add fun into the training as well.

Aside from playing sports, another way to increase stamina is by using an obstacle course. The obstacle course can be a fun and creative way to increase stamina. Very few athletes really enjoy stamina training, but most enjoy the variety and challenge of the obstacle course. This is a good way to spice up the training and improve coordination and strength, too. If possible, set up the obstacle courses in different terrains. This will help the athlete adjust to different topography as well as limiting the chances of becoming easily bored or distracted. Another good option is running on a mountain trail because of the constant change in terrain, hills, slopes, shade, and sun. This all adds to diversity which is always a benefit.

The exercises below are great for building stamina while having fun.

• Quick sprints. Start at one end of a basketball court and sprint to the foul shot line, then back to the original line, and then to the half court line, and back to the original line, then all the way to the other foul shot line and back to the original line, and finally sprint to the other end of the basketball court and back to the original line, which is the other end. Perform two sets at full speed.

• Cone obstacle course. Set 10 cones or obstacles in a zigzag formation one yard apart from each other. Run back and forth, zigzagging through the obstacle course. Perform five times, sprinting at full speed.

• Cone jump. Set five cones or very small boxes in a straight line three yards apart. Sprint while jumping over the boxes. Perform five jumping sprints.

• Track run. Place six cones evenly around a track. Sprint until you arrive at the first cone, then jog until you arrive to the next cone, then sprint again, and so on. Your lap around the track will be alternating sprints and jogs. Perform three laps with a two-minute rest in between.

• Up and down track run. Run three laps around the track and up and down the seating bleachers. Running on the bleachers will provide you with an added level of stamina. Perform three laps.

- Stop watch track run. As you run around the track, do 15-second sprint intervals every minute. Perform three laps.
- Hurdle track run. Run around the track while jumping four small hurdles placed at equal distances around the track. Perform two or three laps.
- Calisthenics track run. Run around the track and, at every halfway point, stop and do 20 push-ups and 20 sit-ups. Perform one to two laps.
- Backward track run. Run backward around the track at a slow pace; as you become comfortable running backward, speed up the pace. Perform 1 lap.
- Water running. This exercise is done in a pool. Stand in the pool at a depth that is up to your thighs. Run in place for 60 seconds. Repeat five times, resting for 10 seconds in between. Then run at a slower pace for 15 straight minutes. Perform one complete set, including five 60-second sprints and one 15 minute jog.
- Ultimate Frisbee. This game is played either 3-on-3 or up to 7-on-7. It's played on a football field but using only half of it. The game follows the same rules as football but with only two downs instead of four and without kicking field goals. Play one game for 30 minutes.

These are just a few examples of different exercises that kids can do to increase their stamina. As the child ages, the intensity and duration of the exercise increases. After a while you will start to see which types of exercises work most effectively for increasing stamina.

There are many types of kids, each one with different fitness goals, different family lifestyles, and different types of bodies and genetics. The truth is that there are many ways for a child to get into shape. The most crucial part of the child's success in achieving the body and health of his or her dreams is the format and presentation of the exercise and diet routine. You can never force a child to eat in a certain way nor can you only offer one or two training regimens. True success will be achieved by constructing a customized meal plan and training routine that the child likes best. You must really focus on making it as fun as possible for the child to get into shape. There are so many food choices and different exercise routines, that at least one of them is bound to interest the child. As a parent, try to focus on this, to shop for the healthiest foods that the child enjoys and will more likely follow. Let us never forget that being healthy is a long-term commitment. Kids like to have fun, so why not have fun with them while getting into shape? The results will come faster and are longer-lasting this way.

23: Increasing Strength

When you are in the early process of learning a particular sport or exercise technique, the golden rule is always "technique over strength." What this means is that before you apply physical strength while performing an exercise or move in sports, is absolutely necessary to perform the drill or exercise many times without weight or force. This will allow you to properly learn the particular move or exercise technique fully before executing it in a real-life situation. Practice the movement over and over again until it is mastered and becomes second nature. If you choose to apply force prior to mastering the move or technique, you will most likely sustain an injury and you will definitely use more energy; hence, you will become tired more quickly.

Kids naturally develop functional strength through their participation in regular activities and sports. Athletes between the ages of 8 and 12 will see faster results and success with their athletic movements and performance rather than with their strength. This is mainly because, until puberty occurs, muscle strength develops at a much lower rate than after puberty. This doesn't mean that strength training should be ignored. Instead, use different strength-enhancing techniques for different age groups. Unfortunately, when people think of strength training they automatically associate it with weight training. There are many other methods that increase strength for kids other than weight training. For kids, weight training should be done sparingly unless the child actively enjoys it. I believe that fun techniques to develop strength for kids should be the primary objective. Kids want to have fun and may lack the discipline of a teenager or adult. The last thing that we would want is to force a child to weight train if he or she doesn't want to, because all this will do is make the child associate fitness with hard work that isn't fun. I personally like having kids perform body-weight calisthenics such as push-ups, pull-ups and free squats for strength exercises. These exercises develop more core strengthening and coordination than weight training, which are key components to excelling in sports and reducing chances of sustaining injury. The real technique is devising the strength-training routine that best suits the individual child and the one that is likely to be enjoyed most.

For athletes from 8 to 12 years old, it is good to focus primarily on continuing the development of natural strength through simple drills to support basic movements that are performed while playing sports. Most of this type of strength training occurs during play. Kids will always naturally develop strength when they engage in sports. It is also a good idea to mix in, from time to time, fun strength-training competitions and drills into other forms of training and games, such as obstacle courses. Doing so deemphasizes the overall stress that strength training can place on a young body and allows for a more diverse training experience.

As children mature from 12 years old and older, their training will involve more weight-training routines. After the age of 12, athletes should gradually accustom themselves more to the use of free weights. Strength training should support and enhance all of the athlete's movement training, meaning agility, balance, coordination, flexibility, speed, and stamina. Weight training, if applied for athletic enhancement, should not be used primarily to build body mass and personal bests in bench pressing and squats, or even dead lifts. This can lead to a focus on how big or defined they can become, rather than developing themselves as athletes and enhancing their sports skills.

Weight training should also be supplemented with continually changing creative play options to keep training experience fresh. Weight training, just like any other activity, must be properly and carefully performed to avoid injury. It is important to make sure the child is properly monitored and properly taught how to correctly weight train. Bad habits early on can develop very quickly and they can lead to injury, improper development of the muscles, and awkward coordination, just to name a few.

The drills below work separate muscle groups throughout the body, with no focus placed on a particular body part or region. For this age group, this method best develops the strength of the child for various sports and athletic functions. Every drill and competition plays an important role in preparing and strengthening the body to move with increased effectiveness and explosive strength.

• Forward and backward crawls. Place two cones a few yards apart for the first course; place four cones in a square formation three to four yards apart for the second course. Crawl forward and backward on hands and knees with the torso facing the ground. On the first course, go back and forth from one cone to the next as many times as possible without falling down. On the square-shaped second course, crawl upside down, with the torso facing the sky. Do as many laps around the four cones as you can without falling down. Perform four sets on the first course and four sets on the second course. Each set ends when you fall over! This exercise improves strength in the arms, shoulders, legs, and core.

• Lateral bench jumps. Place both feet on one side of a bench with one hand placed on each side of the bench. Leap nonstop from one side of the bench to the other ten times. The arms should be locked at the elbows and the knees slightly bent as they travel back and forth over the bench. After 10 repetitions, rest for one minute and then perform another set of 10, for four or five repetitions. Over time, build up to 15 or more reps per set. The bench should be 12 to 18 inches high and 8 to 12 feet long. This exercise should be performed on a stable surface. It strengthens the shoulders and hip flexors as well as overall core strength.

• Medicine ball throws. Using a medicine ball (a large, weighted ball) is a great way to strengthen the body for all types of throwing, swinging, and rotating motions. This is a total body-strength drill that develops the shoulders, arms, legs, and core. Using a lightweight medicine ball, throw the ball as far as you can in a variety of ways: by throwing the ball to each of your sides, throwing it over your head and behind you, and finally throwing it directly in front of you. Perform this exercise 10 times in each of the directions: the sides, rear and front.

• Medicine ball run. Run once around the track holding a medicine ball above your head. This exercise will strengthen your core and shoulders as well as improve stamina.

• Basketball drill. Stand five feet away from a wall. Continuously throw a basketball against the wall and catch it. Try to launch the ball as high up on the wall as possible. Start with a basketball and if you feel comfortable enough, switch to a medicine ball. This exercise strengthens the shoulders and core. Perform 50 repetitions.

Bodyweight Calisthenics

These exercises are performed to increase overall strength.

• Chest: push-ups; incline and decline push-ups; dips. Do five sets of 20 repetitions per exercise.

• Back: pull-ups, close-grip and wide-grip; chin-ups (palms facing you). Do five sets of 10 repetitions per exercise.

• Shoulders: handstand body presses (have someone hold your legs up while you are in a hand-stand position and push yourself up). Perform five sets of 10 repetitions

• Legs: walking lunges; body squats; calf raises. Perform five sets and 20 repetitions of each exercise.

• Neck: lying neck raises (lie on your back and move your head up and down). Perform 100 repetitions.

• Forearms: tennis ball squeeze (continuously squeeze a tennis ball for 2 straight minutes for each arm).

• Biceps: chin-ups (palms facing you). Perform five sets of 10 repetitions.

• Triceps: diamond push-ups (push-ups with your hands placed next to each other without any space in between them). Perform 10 sets of 15 repetitions.

• Abs (lower): leg raises. Perform 50 leg raises while lying flat on your back.

• Abs (upper): crunches. Perform 50 crunches with your elbows touching your thighs.

• Lower back: "Superman" exercise; lie on your stomach with your arms extended in front of your body. Lift your arms and legs while maintaining a straight posture. Perform 20 repetitions.

24: Maximum Speed

Speed is defined as the rate at which athletes move and react to a situation that causes them to change direction. Speed is also a form of reflex and reaction. It doesn't just come from the body but from the mind as well. The time that it takes for your mind to tell your body to perform a particular movement is another basis for speed. Reaction time, reflexes, and physical body speed are all components of speed. Another factor that helps increase speed is flexibility. Being flexible allows your body to have a greater range of motion and requires less energy to move your body, thus allowing your body to operate more efficiently. Speed is an extremely important part of an athlete's success. There is a saying in sports that says, "Power thrills but speed kills." This statement means, that as important as power is, speed is even more important. However, power contributes to speed, along with flexibility and cognitive brain function.

Speed is equally important in every sport, but it is executed in different ways. Depending on the sport, a kid may need to achieve maximum speed for shorter or longer distances or be able to hold maximum speed for longer amounts of time. Some may be starting from a stationary position and others from a moving position. They may have to react to different situations as quickly as possible. Rarely is speed used in only one direction. Often it's paired with a rapid change in direction and incorporates agility.

Speed can be measured in many ways: the speed of movement, or the time it takes to cover a specific distance, or the speed of reaction, or how quickly one can respond to a specific reaction such as a sound, visual image, or touch.

First we will work on how to develop a young athlete's overall running and reaction speed, and then we will work on how to apply speed of reaction to numerous athletic functions.   Nearly all kids, whether they are naturally fast or not, can improve their speed, and this improvement almost always leads to improved all-around athletic performance. To improve a young kid's speed, we must first teach the proper running techniques. Proper running form and overall performance efficiency are essential for improving speed. Once a child learns to run properly, he or she will have more energy and stamina during games or competitions.

One of the most neglected elements in running is proper arm movement. Young athletes often run with their arms just swinging side to side, with no form or synchronicity. Watch a kid's basketball or soccer game and you will see the players run with their arms across their bodies, elbows pointing to each side. Instead of relaxed, cupped hands, you might see something like a full windmill, arms rotating like airplane propellers. But the kids are not to blame for running this way because they have never been taught the proper way. The good news is that it is never too late to learn how to run properly. Once the kids are taught better technique, they begin to experience faster overall running times and increased stamina as a result of reduced energy waste. Proper running technique improves overall athletic efficiency. Practically every athlete can improve their running, even though they may not even notice any flaws.. This is why good coaching is so important for young athletes. A coach monitors the child and improve his or her running and athletic technique.

The form-running drills that I am about to teach you will guide the child-athlete through a series of exercises that focus on one body part at a time. The purpose is to develop muscle memory in each muscle or muscle group before combining the parts. I also include several individual competitions so that the young athlete can self-measure his or her overall progress. The different athletic components such as agility, strength, and balance are interrelated; you can't develop one without developing the other.

Aside from learning how to properly run forward, it is also important for the athlete to know how to run backward efficiently and correctly. During athletic competitions or games, young athletes may need to run backward, and the speed at which they do so may be the difference between a win or a loss. As with form running, it is important to practice the proper techniques of running backward. Unlike regular straight-form running, athletes don't stand straight up when running backward. If they did, they would most likely fall down. The proper posture for running backward is with the waist slightly bent and the shoulders positioned over the knees. The head should always be looking forward. When running backward, it is also important to know how quickly to transition, to "explode" into another direction. Athletes will often switch position from running backward to a full forward run in order to chase an opponent or the ball. For example, when a football cornerback is running backward as the offensive wide receiver approaches to catch the ball, the cornerback must quickly change the position of his hips to change direction into a forward run, so that he can effectively either chase down the wide receiver with the ball or try to catch an interception. These back-and-forth running situations occur in almost every sport.

When I competed in wrestling and boxing, often I would have to execute forward offensive moves and techniques and punches while back-pedaling. The transition from back-pedaling to running is crucial because of the importance of not losing even a step on your opponent or the possibility of regaining possession of the ball. It is the initial pivot and move that are extremely important and should be practiced. This is a great example of how speed and agility skills combine in order to fully execute the most effective movements in athletic competition. Pivoting from backward to forward running is a common quick-execution movement in many sports. Though every sport has different techniques for the transitioning from backward to forward running, I will list a few basic movements and drills that will improve the kid's pivotal movement while playing sports.

Proper form should always be used regardless of the athletic situation to minimize or eliminate all wasted movement and maximize full range of motion as quickly as possible. The transition from one body movement to the next should occur as quickly and smoothly as possible. Playing sports involves frequent stops and starts, changes of direction, all while maneuvering around your opponent as quickly as possible. The speed of an athlete must recover immediately by getting back up as quickly as possible to continue playing while barely missing playing time. Young athletes are often asked to perform these moves during a game or competition without the advantage of practicing and preparing the body's muscle memory to take over and lead the body when it is time to execute the particular move. Kids who play and compete in sports should practice movement changes. The drills and exercises that I list below will provide a great base develop overall running and reactive speed.

Eating for Speed

Proper nutrition plays a vital part in speed. Speed originates from reaction time, which comes from reflex time, and reflex time is determined by relaying a message to the brain. The brain executes the decision, then comes the movement. This entire process is better explained with the example of when you accidentally touch something hot: Your hand automatically jumps back very quickly to avoid the hot surface. As soon as your finger touches the hot surface, a message quickly travels from the finger to the brain, informing the brain that the surface is too hot and to move the finger away from the hot surface. This entire process is known as reflex time.

When the blood is too thick, the message takes longer to travel to the brain and when the brain is inflamed, the neurons won't work as well and as quickly. How can we thin the blood and take away the brain's inflammation? Through exercise and proper nutrition. Exercise forces blood to flow and the brain to make rapid decisions which will make reaction time faster. However, eating properly will do even more to help that process. To thin the blood, a diet of high fiber, monounsaturated and polyunsaturated fats helps keep the arteries smooth and open, allowing the blood to travel faster throughout the body. Eating plenty of fish, olive oil, and nuts and drinking plenty of water will reduce inflammation in the brain. This simple adjustment renders huge benefits that improves cognitive function, mental sharpness, reaction time, speed, and agility. You will notice that after most every workout you will feel mentally sharp and physically agile, because, the blood is rapidly flowing through the body. Your reflex and reaction times improve. It really is a fantastic feeling to be firing on all cylinders. Imagine the mental sharpness that you will have when you combine exercise with proper nutrition. You will really feel that you are on your A game!

Form Running Drill

This exercise will increase speed as well as improve form and technique. Without the proper running form, athletes will never reach their fastest potential running speed. Proper running form allows athletes to eliminate wasted movement, become more efficient, and travel faster in different directions.

Six elements make up an athlete's running form: arm movement, high knees, butt kicks, straight legs, bounding, and rapid leg turnover. This drill progressively works on each of these elements.

• Arm movement. Walk in a straight line for 25 yards, concentrating on marching with arms bent 45 degrees at the elbows. The shoulder, not the elbow, should initiate the arm swing. The arms swing with elbows positioned as close to the body as possible, moving in a straight line, forward and back. The arms should never cross in front of the body. The hands should be gently cupped and relaxed, not clenched or flat, with fingers straight. This prevents the arms from tightening and losing their full range of motion during the arm swing. As the child marches forward, his hands and upper torso should remain as still as possible with shoulders back, not hunched forward. Perform three sets.

- High knees. After the child masters proper arm movement, perform four 25-yard marches while incorporating high knees. This drill exaggerates lifting the knees in comparison to a normal running stride. It trains runners to drive their bodies forward. This exercise activates and stretches the hip flexors, which add to more overall speed. It is important to perform this exercise by lifting the knee as close to the chest as possible. When lowering the leg, it's best for the heel to touch the ground with the toes pointed upward in order to increase flexibility and stride. Perform these strides slowly but with rapid knee lifts. Perform four 25-yard walks and four 25-yard jogs; do four sets of each.
- Butt kicks. This is another exaggerated motion that trains the legs to complete the full range of motion during a running stride. It is important to train and improve the rear part of the running stride. A runner can't reach his maximum speed without getting his back heels as high as possible. This movement isolates, replicates, and exaggerates the movement in order to create muscle memory when all the steps of the running form are put together. Try to have the heels touch the butt, but if not, try to get them as high up as possible. Complete four 25-yard jogs while trying to kick the heels into the butt. Try to drive each leg back to the ground rapidly after touching your butt, causing the feet to pull the ground backward as the body explodes forward. Try to feel your toes pulling toward the shins each time your feet contact the ground, because this will engage the calf muscle and help push the body forward by pushing against the ground. The positioning of the toes toward the shin on each stride pulls each foot through faster, increasing running speed. Perform four 25-yard sets.
- Straight leg. This exercise is performed by walking in a straight line while keeping your legs completely straight and pointing toes upward. Keeping the toes up allows the feet to get up faster off the ground, increasing speed and flexibility. Keeping the toes up while lowering the foot quickly to the ground is how the counter-force is produced—and counter-force is what generates the speed. Perform three 30-yard walks and three 25-yard jogs. When transitioning from a walk to a jog,

you will begin to feel a greater backward pulling force on each foot. Perform three sets of 25 yards walking and three of 25 yards jogging.

• Leaping. This exercise strengthens the body's ability to explode forward and strengthens the body. The best way to explain this drill is to think of jumping over puddles of water with long, leaping jumps. With each jump, drive forward with the right knee while using the left leg (with the toes up) to thrust off the ground for distance. Land on the right foot and immediately thrust off the ground with the same foot (toes up), this time driving the left knee forward. This continues throughout the exercise. Perform fur sets of 25-yard non-stop leaps.

• Backward speed drill races. Do a backward running race. Make sure the kids are looking straight ahead, not down. The body should have a slight bend and the feet should be close together and underneath the body. Smaller sets will provide better balance when racing. The race should be performed in a straight line. Perform four races of 25 yards.

• Change of direction. You will need a whistle for this exercise. Place four cones in a square formation approximately 10 yards apart from each other. Have the kids sprint from one cone to the next, using the whistle to determine which cone to run to. For example, one whistle blow means sprint to cone #1, two whistle blows: sprint to cone #2, three blows: #3, and four blows: #4. Each time the whistle blows, the child changes direction and sprints to the correct cone. This drill will effectively increase split-second direction change time. Perform six sets with the 4-whistle blows.

• Multiple speed moves. This exercise will increase the athlete's speed when changing direction from a lateral to a forward movement. You will need a whistle for this exercise. Begin by having the athlete jog in a forward motion. After 20 seconds, blow the whistle once, which signals the athlete to sprint forward for 20 seconds; blow the whistle again, signaling the athlete to jog again. Blow it twice for the athlete to begin jogging to the left side for 20 seconds, then blow again for the athlete to return to the jogging forward motion. Blow three times, which means for the athlete to begin laterally jogging to the right, with a shuffle, then blow again, but this time signaling the athlete to sprint forward for 20 seconds. Finally blow the whistle four times, signaling the athlete to begin to backward jog for 20 seconds until the whistle is blown again, which would then have the athlete switch to a 20-second forward sprint. Perform four sets.

• Slalom dash. Set up six cones or objects on the ground, placing them in a straight line 10 yards apart. Have the kid sprint around each cone, touching them near the bottom after passing them. After every two cones, switch directions and sprint forward. Do two cones for the first set, then four cones for the second set, then finally six cones for the last set. Be sure to always touch the bottom of the cone in order to improve core flexibility and overall agility. Perform four sets.

• Speed change obstacle course. Fr this exercise you will need to set a 30-yard obstacle course with cones and boxes. Set up a cone or box every five yards in a zigzag formation. Sprint around every cone while touching the bottom of the cone without stopping and jump over every box at a full sprint. Run around this obstacle course at least five times, with explosive speed. Perform five to seven sets.

• Lying down drills. To perform this exercise you will need two cones or other objects and a stopwatch. Set up the two cones or objects as a starting and finishing point 25 yards apart from each other. Start at the first cone or object from several different positions: lying face down, lying face up, sitting cross-legged facing forward, and sitting cross-legged facing backward When the whistle blows, the kid must get to his feet as quickly as possible and sprint to the next cone or object. As each set passes, try to achieve faster times. Perform four sets from each starting position, with a 20-second rest time between exercises. This exercise helps strengthen and activate core muscles.

• Wrestler's stance exercise. This exercise is specialized for wrestlers and football players. The drill involves squatting with the back vertical and the thighs horizontal. The first part of the exercise involves walking in each of the four directions while in this position. The second part involves sprinting in that position in each of the four directions for

20-second bursts. This exercise will stretch and strengthen the hamstrings as well as the lower back muscles. Perform four sets of 20-second sprints in each position.

• Basketball speed drill. This drill involves running on a basketball court while dribbling the ball. You will develop speed, agility, and real game-like movements. Perform this drill by setting up nine or 10 cones or other objects on the court in a straight line. Sprint from one end of the court to the other while dribbling the basketball from one hand to the other. Perform seven sets. Each set includes sprinting from one side to the other while zigzagging through the cones or objects.

25: Improving Agility

Athletes with agility are usually quick and flexible and have a combination of mental sharpness, alertness, and intelligence as well as good cognitive function. Agility is what makes an athlete move so gracefully while playing the sport. A boxer relies on agility to avoid punches and execute punches from all angles. A tennis player uses agility to hit the tennis ball while running. A wide receiver uses agility to catch a pass while leaping into the air. Every athlete needs agility to be competitive.

Training for agility is about training for body awareness and creating rhythm in the athlete's movements. The more aware they are of how their bodies feel when executing different movements at different speeds, the more success they will have in competition. This feel is also called muscle memory, which is an actual rhythm that the body creates to remember and react under different circumstances. Think of a young athlete playing in a basketball game. There are so many combinations of body movements that occur during the game, from stop-and-go running, to cutting with one foot in one direction and immediately cutting back with the other foot, to running with the ball, to passing to receive the ball, all while moving at different speeds in one smooth transition. Agility and coordination are similarly related, and agility training is an important part to developing coordination. Think of sport-specific coordination skills such as a basketball player shooting a basket while running, a volleyball player saving a ball while diving, and a lacrosse player catching a pass and quickly re-passing the ball while on the run. None of these plays would be possible if the athletes had not improved their agility. As they develop their agility skills, they are also improving their muscle memory and body awareness. Athletes who have good agility don't have to think about what they are doing because, with muscle memory, the body naturally falls into the right position and the right place.

A boxer doesn't have to think before ducking to avoid a punch. This movement occurs automatically through hours of training which develops muscle memory. Agility training prepares the body to react and become comfortable moving in the most effective and efficient ways possible to make important plays and improve overall performance. All different body movements, both upper and lower, either separate or synchronized, become second nature with agility training. The best of athletes cannot improve without continually developing this important trait. Some trainers combine agility training with conditioning. but I do not suggest this. Agility drills are extra important; they need individualized attention. After agility training, athletes can then incorporate other elements such as conditioning into their regimen. For example, after hours of specific agility training, passing a soccer ball on the run or passing a football while being rushed by several defenders, becomes a simple progression. The sooner young athletes begin agility training, the faster they will see the overall improvement in their performance. Of all the different elements of being an athlete, agility should be the most enjoyable for kids to learn because it allows for creativity, which kids really enjoy. No one athlete moves exactly the same as the other, so every one of them must find their own most effective way to move. Agility training allows young athletes to develop their own style in relation to their body type, developing abilities, and genetics. They must discover their gift, natural movement, or style that they feel most comfortable with and which best suits their body type. Every athlete will have that one move that he or she loves and is good at. He or she should work hard on improving and perfecting it.

Agility Drills
• Blind-folded jump rope. This exercise develops muscle memory and

agility. Perform this exercise by first jumping rope with your eyes open and face uncovered. Then, for the second part of the exercise, begin to jump rope while blindfolded. Perform three three-minute rounds with eyes open and four three-minute rounds while blindfolded.

• Multi-level sprint. This exercise develops agility while your body is constantly changing levels. Perform this exercise by placing six hurdles in a straight line 10 yards apart. Begin by sprinting to leap over one hurdle and crawling under the next for one set, then crawling under all six hurdles for the next set, and jumping over all six hurdles for the last set. Perform two sets of drill.

• Ball passing sprint. This drill improves both agility and eye-hand coordination. Perform this exercise on an outdoor field 30 yards long and with a football, a soccer ball, and a tennis ball. Begin by running on the field while the trainer throws you the football and pass it back to him all while running. Do the same with a tennis ball; try to catch the ball with the same hand that you throw with. Finally, the trainer foot-passes the soccer ball while the athlete passes back the ball while running. Perform three sets of each exercise.

• Multi-movement body drill. In most sports it is important to be able to adjust your body from any position. Movement often comes suddenly, including being hit and falling to the ground. Regardless of the situation, we must be able to quickly get back into position and form. For this exercise you will need three small boxes or hurdles, a cushioned mat, and eight cones or objects. Place one cone at the starting point, another cone five yards in front, another cone five yards in front of the previous cone. Then place the mat in front of the third cone just two to three yards from the cone. After the mat, place the three small boxes or hurdles that are to be jumped, followed by five cones each five yards apart. Perform this exercise as if you were on an obstacle course and are attempting to improve your time. Begin by sprinting to the first cone and circling it, then sprinting to the second, and then to the third cone. After the third cone, do forward rolls on the tumbling mat and then jump the three small hurdles. Finish off the obstacle course by sprinting and circling around the remaining five cones. During each drill, work toward improving your time. This exercise will improve agility and explosiveness. Perform five sets of this exercise, each set is one completion of the obstacle course.

• Swap meet. This exercise is performed by jumping up onto a bench that is 12 inches high. It is done to increase agility in different positions off of explosive body movements. Begin this drill by standing two feet away from a 12-inch-high bench. While standing in front of the bench, jump onto the bench by lifting both feet at the same time for the first set. For the second set, start by standing on the bench and jumping back downward. For the third set, jump onto the bench and back to the ground without stopping. On the fourth set, stand on the bench backward and jump onto the floor, landing forward. For this set you will perform a 180-degree turn while in the air. For the last set, face opposite the bench, jumping onto it and landing in a forward position. Again you will be twisting your body in midair. Perform four sets of this exercise. Each set includes jumping in five different movements onto the bench. Work to increase your speed for each set.

• Fast feet drill. This exercise will develop coordination while taking small steps in a shuffling motion. You will need a rope ladder or regular ladder that is at least 12 feet in length. Lay the ladder on the ground. Begin by running the length of the ladder as quickly as possible, placing your feet in each of the spaces in between its rungs. Begin this exercise by running forward as quickly as possible, while making sure not to miss any rungs. The next variation includes running backward, while not missing any rungs. The third variation includes running sideways while shuffling your feet; perform this exercise running on both sides, both left and right. The final variation includes running the length of each side of the ladder with one foot running inside the rung spaces and the other foot running outside. Perform five total sets. Each set includes all variations.

• Side shuffle crossover run. This exercise involves running to the side while crossing the legs. This drill will improve both lateral and overall agility. Begin these drills by running sideways 30 yards to the left and then 30 yards to the right. While running to either side, feet and legs must cross over each other in order to achieve the maximum step distance and stretch. This drill will loosen the hip flexors and improve agility. Perform 10 total sets. Each set includes running to each side of the body.

• Sports specific obstacle course. This exercise involves running through an obstacle course with different athletic equipment such as a Frisbee, football, soccer ball, football, baseball, and tennis or racquet ball. Place one item 10 yards apart from each other in a line. Begin by doing 50 push-ups and 50 sit-ups. When finished, sprint 10 yards to the Frisbee, then and drop to the ground and perform 10 push-ups and 10 sit-ups. Next, immediately throw the Frisbee as far and accurately as you can. After the Frisbee, sprint to the basketball, perform the push-ups and sit-ups, then dribble the basketball in each hand. Next, sprint toward the football and after completing the calisthenics, throw the football as hard and as far as you can. Next sprint to the soccer ball and, after performing the calisthenics, try to foot dribble the soccer ball for as long as possible. Sprint to the baseball, and after performing the calisthenics, hit the ball as far and as hard as possible. Finally, do the same when sprinting towards the tennis or racquet ball. After performing the calisthenics, hit the ball with either the tennis or racquet ball racquet as far as possible. Perform two sets. Each set includes performing all of the actions and exercises. This exercise will increase sports-specific agility.

• Sports specific calisthenics drill. This exercise increases agility and strengthens the body's core. This exercise involves using a basketball, soccer ball, and football. Begin this exercise by performing 10 push-ups, followed by 10 sit-ups and 10 jumping squats. Once the calisthenics are completed, immediately shoot the basketball 10 times into the basket without stopping. Next, perform the same calisthenics, followed by throwing the football 10 consecutive times. The last exercise will include performing the calisthenics followed by foot-juggling the soccer ball, then kicking it as far as possible. Perform 10 sets. Each set includes all three exercises.

These exercises are for the advanced young athlete. All will improve all parts of the athlete's requirements for speed, agility, balance, strength, stamina, and coordination. The child will notice the difference even by his or her walk and, of course, athletic performance. Constant practice will bring steady improvement every step of the way.

26: Improving Throwing and Kicking

Growing up, I can remember how amazed I was when another child really had a powerful throwing arm, the person who could really blast that football down the field, or that baseball player who threw the baseball as if his arm was a cannon, or when playing soccer, that one particular player who had such firepower in his leg that whenever the soccer ball was kicked it seemed as if the ball would explode. I remember saying to myself, "How could I throw or kick like that?" Along with power, accuracy is important as well. In order to be able to throw an accurate baseball you must first point the opposite throwing shoulder directly toward the designated target. The throwing arm must keep the elbow above the shoulder. The most common and effective throwing technique is the "throwing over the top" technique. This technique provides the most power and accuracy. Foot position is very important as well because a large part of the throwing power originates from the feet and how they are positioned. When throwing, the front foot should be well planted to the ground while the rear foot must be used for pushing off of the ball of the foot. When throwing a baseball using full power, the body must twist with the majority of force coming from the rear foot pushing forward. Throwing the football is a little different because, for one, the ball is much larger; the hand must grab the ball with the fingers spread over the laces and index finger extended toward the tip of the ball. Proper throwing position starts by placing the feet shoulder width apart and the opposite shoulder pointed toward the direction of the throw. The football pass begins by bringing the football all the way toward the back of the ear, and with the back of the ball pointed in a straight line and slightly behind the thrower's body. Right before the ball is thrown, the body weight is shifted onto the rear foot. When throwing the ball, the lower body moves first, shifting the body weight from the back foot to the front foot with the hips and shoulders following and squaring up with the front foot. The non-throwing arm is released from the football and keeps moving around the body, while pulling the throwing arm through. The throwing arm follows the ball as it leaves the hand with the index finger pointing in the direction of the target and palm facing the ground. Throwing a lacrosse ball is similar to throwing a baseball. The shoulders remain perpendicular to the target as the athlete points the opposite shoulder at the target. Begin throwing by placing the top hand near the head of the stick, then throw with the top hand, pull with the bottom hand, and step with the front foot toward the target. The athlete follows through with the stick, finishing with the head pointing toward the target and the stick parallel to the ground. Usually, the top hand is the dominant throwing hand.

Kicking a soccer ball with force has a lot to do with balance as well. However, resistance leg training will help increase the force of the kick. Practicing proper form running is important, not just to increase speed while running, but improve the power of the kick. In reality, a strong kick works in tandem with speed while running, in other words, in order to develop a powerful kick it is important to develop speed while running. Powerful legs also need to be stretched. Previously I wrote about the various ways to increase running speed. This should be applied to kicking also. Stretching all of the leg muscles is very important. Begin kicking by placing the opposite foot fast in the direction of the target. While getting a slight running start, plant the foot next to the ball and pointed toward the target. While pulling the kicking leg back lean slightly forward and drive the leg forward and kick the ball while remaining in a slightly bent forward formation. Another great method of increasing kicking strength is tying an elastic band around the kicking ankle while the end of the elastic is tied to a fixed object slightly behind, and practice swinging the leg in a kicking formation but without the ball. The resistance will strengthen the power of the kick.

Whether it is a boxer's punch, a soccer player's kick, a baseball player's bat swing, or a football quarterback's throw, all of these actions will always work more effectively and with more success if they are performed with more power and accuracy. Power and speed work together simultaneously. Therefore, it is always best to work on both, because when both speed and power are combined, it equals a recipe for success.

27: Fitness for Teenagers

Fitness for a teenager varies quite a bit from that of a child. A teenager is now beginning to realize the shape of his body, and the specific sports that he or she wants to play. Another difference between the teenager and child is that children are less focused on what sport they want to play and what body type they want have; they have more of a free-spirited, live-for-the-moment attitude and approach. In contrast, teenagers begin to be more conscious about themselves and take necessary steps in order to gain that feeling of self-worth and acceptance. These steps to gain social acceptance usually mean achieving some type of success. The success could mean being a great athlete, having a great body, being a scholar, or even being the best at computer games; basically, any type of fame among their peers which would most likely come from any type of success. The point is that the psychology of the teenager changes drastically from that of the child. Competitiveness begins to set in, which creates a more driven mentality.

The mistake many teenagers make is the same mistake that I made when I was that age. I didn't educate myself enough to learn how to be that great athlete or that great scholar. I did know that it took some type of commitment but I was still very clueless about the steps I could take to be that successful teenager. Working and preparing with maximum efficiency must be a top priority in your approach toward any type of training.

At this point, you may be asking yourself, how all of this could apply to getting into shape? Efficiency applies to getting into shape because you want the maximum results with the least effort. For example, for a cardiovascular workout, instead of walking on a treadmill (which you may not enjoy doing), play a game of handball instead. Another example of efficiency is when preparing grilled chicken breast and sweet potato. Why not grill three pieces of chicken breast at once and microwave three sweet potatoes at once? Because for nearly the same amount of time and effort you now have three meals instead of one. That's called efficiency! One last example of improving efficiency: Imagine going for a three-mile jog that may take 30 minutes to complete. Instead of the jog, perform 10 50-yard sprints, each sprint performed every minute, which gives you a full cardiovascular workout in 10 minutes as opposed to 30 minutes for the job.

The success of any type of fitness always begins with the psychology behind it all. You must think properly to effectively execute the components that will enable you to achieve all your fitness goals. Teenagers are looking for great results in the fastest time possible. Teenagers also have more physical capacity to endure demanding workouts. Kids in this age group have so much more social pressures to succeed. This pressure comes from themselves, their parents and coaches, and their peers. Teenagers may feel overwhelmed by this. They may doubt their abilities, but in reality, the fear mainly comes from not knowing how to exercise and eat.

28: Stretching

For years, people that I have trained, and fellow athletes that I competed with, have asked me about stretching. Stretching comes to everyone's mind as something healthy, something it's important to do before and after every workout to improve the workout and avoid injury. This actually isn't true at all. Stretching can sometimes be an unnatural movement that could even be unsafe or counter-productive. We have all heard that stretching is so good for us that it has become practically written in stone. The truth is that there is really no such thing as muscular flexibility. Muscles are made up of groups of fibers that contract (shorten) and lengthen as the joint flexes and extends. Joints possess flexibility, while muscles possess contractility. Performing stretching exercises to make the muscle more flexible is like pulling on a door to make it open wider. If you pull the door hard enough, you will end up damaging the door's hinges and maybe even the door itself. But then why is it that people, after a stretch, seemingly move their joints throughout a greater range of motion? Researchers have looked at this and have found that when people engage in stretching programs, the contractile properties of the muscle do not change. This means the muscles don't receive any benefit. What happened was the people in these studies only became more tolerant of the pain that came from stretching. You can try this out for yourself. Sit on the floor and straighten out your legs to the front of your body. Sit up as tall as possible and slowly, while keeping your back arched and rigid, try to touch your toes. As you stretch farther and farther, you'll soon feel pain in the back of your thighs. Don't push past this point. If you performed this stretch every day for several weeks, you would eventually get used to the feeling of pain and be able to stretch further. This is called stretch tolerance. That is all that is, just tolerance to pain, tolerance to that stretch. You have not created longer or more pliable muscles. All that you have done is become used to the feeling. Pilates experts and physical therapists agree on this point. I know many coaches and trainers advocate stretching, especially for kids who are involved in sports, and I know it seems as if it is a good thing for kids. Still, there is no scientific evidence or any theoretical basis for stretching. If you stretch too much, you can damage the ligaments that connect the bones together. Ligaments have very little blood flow and when they are stretched and lengthened, they are lengthened permanently! This may be necessary if you are a ballet dancer, but it is definitely not healthy.

Studies have shown that an athlete's power output is decreased when he stretches a lot, as it can loosen ligaments and tendons to the point where less force can be developed, just like an old and worn-out rubber band. If you or your child are involved in a sport that requires explosive power such as wrestling, football, hockey, or sprinting, stretching may be counter-productive.

When kids and teenagers become stronger they become better able to move a joint through a greater range of motion. They can perform any joint motion better because the underlying muscles are better able to move the joint and better able to stabilize and protect joints from injury. Strength training, not stretching, improves joint range of motion in adults and teens. We tend to use the word "stretching" in the wrong context. For example, a child wakes up in the morning and pulls his or her elbows back, thereby stretching the chest muscles. But is the child actually doing this? What happens is that by pulling on the arm muscles, the muscles of the back contract and thus, the muscles of the chest stretch. What the child is doing is squeezing and contracting the muscles in the back. So rather than call this stretching, it should be called contracting. Powerfully contracting your muscles through strength training is the best way to increase muscular strength, which will improve joint flexibility. I bet that you never knew this. I sure didn't for many years. This is why we should let exercise science, and not exercise tradition, guide our health and fitness endeavors. A joint should never be made more flexible without a simultaneous increase in strength in the muscles that surround it. The bottom line is that there is no need to stretch before or after a strength training program or any type of exercise. Stretching to increase safety or to improve athletic performance should be greatly reconsidered.

Having said all this, I am aware that many people still like to stretch and feel good when they do it. If stretching is something that makes you feel good, then by all means do it, but with caution and very lightly. Remember that you do not need to stretch before or after exercising.

Let's not confuse stretching with warming up before exercising. I will use myself as an example. As the competitive athlete that I have always been, I always practiced the art of warming up rather than stretching, prior to engaging in high-intensity activity.

When you warm up, your body simply flows better and your endurance is improved. Warming up includes mild exercise and drilling in exactly the activity that you are about to do, but in a gentle way until you just begin to sweat. Once you begin to sweat, your body is ready for high-intensity activity.

Have you ever watched a boxing match on TV and noticed that the two athletes are walking into the ring already sweating? Or when watching a football game, you'll see the kicker is warming up by practicing kicks on the sidelines. Do you ever see these athletes actually stretching? I have played on many a sports team and before the event started I was always told by the coach to warm up, which meant to loosen up, get the body nice and warm and fluid in its motions.

Do you also know how important it is to warm up before playing to prevent an injury? When the body is cold, the muscles are stiff and brittle, making it more prone to injury. For example, a few years back I arrived late to wrestling practice. All the other wrestlers had already warmed up. One of the wrestlers asked me, "Chris, are you ready for live wrestling or do you need to warm up?" I made the grave mistake of saying, "I'm ready to wrestle." Sure enough, it proved to be disastrous. Within two minutes, I felt such an intense pain in my chest that all I could do was lie there, holding my chest, immobilized. About an hour later, I was able to stand up and be taken to the hospital for treatment. After an MRI scan the doctor had said that I had torn my chest (pectoral) muscle. This injury was attributed to not warming up before going "all out" on the wrestling mat. Huge mistake!

Warming up and breaking a sweat prior to playing sports also increases your endurance. Every time I competed in sports without breaking a sweat before, I also immediately became tired. However, after a good sweat and warm up, I performed much better in the game. This is what athletes call their "second wind." The second wind will last a much longer time because your body is running at full efficiency. Always warm up enough to go out on the field to compete on your "second wind." It is the best way to perform.

29: Warming Up

Warming up is an extremely important preliminary to exercise. The first 15 minutes of any type of exercise always seem like the hardest part of the training session. Every time I exercise, the first 15 minutes aren't fun at all; they're the hardest part. To make the best of those first 15 minutes, I do the exercise with less intensity until I feel fully warmed up. Depending on the exercise, the warm-up varies.

A proper warm-up will really change your workout experience in a very positive. Your experience will go from not wanting to train, to absolutely loving the workout! The warm-up is that important! I am always looking ways to add fun to my training, especially the beginning of the workout, the part I enjoyed the least. I know that going onto the soccer field or wrestling mat on a "second wind" was crucial. I tried many ways to get that second wind as quickly and as enjoyably as possible.

Another motivating factor for warming up is when you begin to feel the psychological benefits of exercise. This is called the "runner's high." Once this state of mind is achieved, all of a sudden the exercise becomes fun, euphoric, and mentally therapeutic. This is the state that you look to achieve during every workout. The runner's high or endorphin rush is the main reason why I work out daily. I look forward to achieving this feeling because it makes the workout feel amazing! This elevated mental state usually last for several hours after the workout finishes.

Let's start with the physical feeling of lifting weights. After numerous sets, the muscles that are being trained become engorged with lactic acid and blood; we call this the "pump." The pump feeling makes the muscle look larger and harder. You feel better mentally because you feel stronger, bigger, and more powerful. The combination of the pump and the endorphin rush is an unbelievable combination that you can experience during every workout. Other sports will give you a similar high. For example, after I play a game of soccer, the endorphin rush is at its best. The physical feeling I experience is that my body feels extremely loose and my skin is glowing. All the sweating clears the pores in your skin, giving you a glowing, radiant, very healthy look. Aside from the mental and physical attributes of exercising, once you are warmed up, it seems that your brain is functioning at its peak for accurate, split-second decisions.

Warming up lets you perform at your best while also enjoying yourself. Fun is the priority. When you enjoy what you are doing, then chances are you will have more success.

Warm-Up Activities

• Soccer. Jog for 10 minutes with an occasional 20-yard sprint every two minutes of jogging. For the next 10 minutes, practice running with the ball, kicking it into a goal, and passing it to other teammates. By this time you should be breaking a sweat.

• Wrestling. Jog around the mat for five minutes. For the next five minutes, practice penetration shots across both ways of the mat. For the following 10 minutes, drill takedowns with your workout partner. Drill without stopping for 10 minutes. Work to tire yourself in order to expand the lungs for increased oxygen intake.

• Tennis. Jog for five minutes with your knees high up. For the next 15 minutes, practice hitting the ball with the racket, using against a wall or with a partner.

• Football. Jog for five minutes. For the following five minutes, practice sprint/jog drills. Sprint until tired, then jog until recuperated, then sprint again. For the last 10 minutes, practice running and passing, side shuffling, and running/sprinting in all different directions.

• Racquetball. For 10 minutes, practice hitting the ball against the wall in all different racket positions, including backhand, traditional, and serving.

• Basketball. Jog for five minutes. For the following five minutes, practice jogging while dribbling. The next five minutes should be dedicated to jogging and shooting the ball and the final five minutes spent practicing team plays.

• Boxing. Jump rope for four three-minute rounds. Shadowbox for three three-minute rounds. Use the speed bag for three three-minute rounds followed by three three-minute rounds with the heavy bag. Focus on speed and accuracy while punching the speed bag and focus on power and balance while hitting the heavy bag.

30: Water

Never could I stress to you enough the importance of drinking enough water. Most people neglect to drink enough water throughout the day, which is not healthy at all. Here's why water is so important to the body:

• Approximately 75 percent of Americans are chronically dehydrated and this most likely applies to half of the world's population.

• In 37 percent of Americans, the thirst mechanism is so weak that it is often mistaken for hunger.

• Even mild hydration will slow down your metabolism by as much as 3 percent.

• One glass of water shuts down the feeling of midnight hunger.

• A lack of water is the main cause of daytime fatigue.

• Preliminary research indicates that drinking eight to 10 glasses of water a day could significantly ease back joint pain for up to 80 percent of sufferers.

• A mere 2 percent drop in body weight can cause fuzzy short-term memory, trouble with basic math, and difficulty focusing on the computer screen or on a printed page.

• Drinking five glasses of water daily decreases the risk of colon cancer by 45 percent. It can slash the risk of breast cancer by 70 percent, and you are 50 percent less likely to develop bladder cancer.

• Your body uses approximately 150 calories to heat a gallon of refrigerated water to 98.6 degrees (body temperature) in order to void it, so if you want to lose fat faster, then drink a lot!

Water and Your Child

How important is water for the teenager and child? Well, consider that our bodies range from 50 to 65 percent water, and some experts say it's even more. Without water we can live for only a few days. As the saying goes, you are what you eat, but you are what you drink as well. Not all body parts have the same amount of water. Here is the basic breakdown:

Blood: 90%

Brain: 85%

Muscle: 75%

Skin: 71%

Bone: 30%

Body fat: 15%

Looks like the body finds water fairly important, no? Clearly, if you don't drink enough water, you will slowly but surely become dehydrated. As your body experiences dehydration, you will more than likely feel it first in those areas that contain most water. For example, at first you will lose alertness and feel fuzzy in your head. Next, you will suffer from total body muscular fatigue. As you can see from the chart, dehydration doesn't affect your fat much. Why is this so important? Well, most of us, and especially overweight kids, need to lose fat. The idea that excessive sweating is good for fat loss makes little sense. In fact, staying cool burns many more calories than keeping warm, and all without the water loss.

Water is actually a type of food. You may not think of it this way, but it's the most important nutritional necessity in your entire eating plan. As I had mentioned before, you can't live very long without it. So that you can visualize the importance of water, here is a short list of the many purposes water serves in your body.

• Acts as a solvent for vitamins, minerals, amino acids, and glucose

• Transports vital nutrients

• Aids in the digestion of food

- Lubricates your joints
- Serves as a type of shock absorber inside the eyes and spinal cord
- Helps regulate and maintain body temperature
- Rids the body of waste products (and fat) through the urine
- Disseminates heat through the skin, lungs, and urine
- Assists in intense muscular contraction

In short, water is vital and critically important aspect of our daily eating regimen. Try using flavored waters that contain no sugar if you have trouble drinking enough plain water.

Warning: Partial Dehydration

If you are aware and sensitive enough to your own and your child's body, you should be able to recognize some of the early warnings of partial dehydration. Here are the symptoms of partial dehydration:

- Dizziness
- Headaches
- Fatigue
- Thirst
- Flushed skin
- Blurred vision
- Muscle weakness

Many people, even sports coaches, wait too long to hydrate, sometimes allowing dehydration symptoms to occur. This is one of the reasons that sports teams use sports drinks such as Gatorade to make water tasty to drink. Offering these tastier alternatives ensures that athletes will more readily remain hydrated. Unfortunately, most people, even athletes, never realize that, most of the time, they are in a state of partial dehydration. In fact, some experts suggest that long before you are thirsty, you are already somewhat dehydrated. To avoid this, have a big drink before starting your activity and take regular water breaks during the activity.

Flushing Out the Fat

Water aids the fat-loss process in many ways. One of the most important is in allowing the internal organs to function properly. For example, your kidneys need sufficient water. If they don't receive it, your liver actually takes over and performs some of the functions of the kidneys. This can short-change your liver's most important task, which is to convert stored fat into fuel. To maximize your metabolism, you must drink plenty of water.

Reducing Appetite

When you lose fat, most of it is lost as heat from your skin. Yep, right off the old epidermis. The two other ways you lose fat is breathing it out and when you urinate. Drinking a gallon of water per day will speed fat loss and improve health. Drinking large amounts of water can double, triple, or even quadruple your urine production. As a result, you will be able to eliminate more heat. Remember, inside your body, fat loss means heat loss. Going to the bathroom so many times a day may be inconvenient, but it offers many health benefits. And the colder the water the better! When you drink cold water, your body has to heat it to your normal body temperature of 98.6 degrees. It takes approximately one calorie to heat one ounce of water to the body's core temperature. So an eight-ounce glass of cold water burns approximately 8 calories. One gallon of cold water burns approximately 128 calories. Another way to help this acclimation is to sip the water instead of gulping it. Using a straw sometimes makes it easier to sip.

Cure for Constipation

Another one of the many functions of water is to help prevent constipation. Super hydration makes bowel movements much easier if this is an issue. There is no need to use stool-softening drugs; use water instead.

Purified Water vs. Tap Water

Many experts claim that most water that comes from the tap, especially in apartment buildings, is tainted. It could be that there is too much metal or too many minerals (perhaps from old building pipes), but unless you have your water professionally tested, you will never be certain of the water's impurities, or if there even are any. The American water supply is very safe and your tap water is probably perfectly fine to drink. If you are concerned about your tap water or if it unusually hard or soft, you can install a reverse osmosis system under the sink. The filter removes minerals and just about everything else from the water, which is both good and bad. I have tried drinking purified spring water, purified tap water, distilled water, and tap water. I prefer tap water. For me it's more convenient, much less expensive (free), and a lot more accessible (any sink). Buying spring water becomes an expense and a hassle when you constantly are carrying heavy gallons home from the store. Why not just open your kitchen faucet to pour yourself a glass of water? I have tried drinking distilled water, but because it is depleted of its minerals, it acts as a diuretic. The diuretic effect helps rid a small amount of excess water retention, giving the body a more defined look. But it often leads to cramps. When I need to give my body a more defined look, I drink nothing but tap water and carefully monitor my food intake. This is a much safer and healthier way to look your best. Throughout the years I am realizing more and more that there are no shortcuts to looking your best. Nothing beats a well-planned diet, having the proper amount of water and food, but most importantly, the proper amount of time to achieve your physical goals.

31: Eat Well, Nature's Medicine

We are all aware of the physical benefits of eating healthy. We all definitely want to look better, but we often forget the other benefits of healthy eating. A healthy diet and exercising by themselves can help reduce the risk of getting a chronic illness such as high cholesterol, high blood pressure, type 2 diabetes, and colon cancer. Basic foods such as olive oil, water, fish, and vegetables will do wonders for your health. I will give you a few examples of how eating right and exercising may help prevent chronic illness or make it easier to handle if it does occur.

High Cholesterol

High cholesterol can make your arteries, especially the arteries that feed the heart, become filled with plaque. Clogged arteries restrict or block the passage of blood, which can lead to strokes and heart attacks. This buildup of plaque is an accumulation of "bad" cholesterol, including LDL (low-density lipoprotein), VLDL (very low density lipoprotein), and triglycerides (tiny fat droplets in your blood). A combination of these three forms of "bad" cholesterol will cause you to have high cholesterol. This illness can be combated by exercising and eating a diet that is low in bad fat and high in good fat. Good fats are olive oil, canola oil, almonds, fish, walnuts, flaxseed, avocado and peanuts. Eating a diet with plenty of these foods will help reduce your total cholesterol. All of the meal plans I construct are laden with all of the necessary foods that will help lower your total cholesterol, blood pressure, and reduce the chances of colon cancer, all at the same time!

High Blood Pressure

High blood pressure is a very common condition. The number of people who suffer from high blood pressure keeps rising because being overweight and eating a diet that is high in salt and refined carbohydrates, along with not exercising, are common causes of high blood pressure. Simply exercising and eating a diet that is high in fiber and low in sodium will most definitely help lower your blood pressure. It is a very important to drink three to four quarts of water per day as well.

Colon Cancer

Colon cancer may be caused by the constant buildup of undigested food that remains in the intestines for extended periods of time. The reason the food remains in the intestines without being digested is due to a lack of fiber in the diet. Fiber and water will speed the food through the digestive tract where enzymes break it down for digestion. The problem today is most people don't eat enough fiber or drink enough water, which may eventually lead to colon cancer. Eating a diet that is rich in vegetables, fruits and whole grains, along with drinking at least two quarts of water per day, may reduce the chances of colon cancer. Try to consume at least 25 to 35 grams of fiber per day.

Type 2 Diabetes

Type 2 diabetes happens when your cells become resistant to the effects of the hormone insulin, which carries glucose (blood sugar) into the cells where it is burned for fuel. Usually, type 2 diabetes is an illness of older adults who are overweight or obese and sedentary. It was rarely seen in younger people, but type 2 diabetes rates have skyrocketed among children and teens in recent years. This is been primarily caused by the drastic increase in sugar consumption, which has led to an epidemic of obesity. Too many sugary foods and drinks raises the blood sugar; the pancreas has to produce lots of extra insulin to deal with the extra sugar. Eventually, the pancreas burns out from the overwork and no longer works efficiently.

Preventing the onset of type 2 diabetes is simple: change your diet to limit sugars and refined carbohydrates. Carbohydrates are desirable following a workout or for breakfast, because at these times the body is depleted of glucose. Eating simple carbohydrates at that point will immediately provide a boost in your blood sugar that your muscles will take up right away. The rest of the time, however, insulin will carry off excess blood sugar to be stored as body fat.

To avoid this serious disease, it is important to eat small portions, especially complex (slow-acting) carbohydrates, frequently throughout the day. Eating every two to four hours will provide the body with a steady stream of energy throughout the day and will limit the chances of developing type 2 diabetes. Complex carbohydrates include brown and wild rice, sweet potatoes, whole-grain pasta, oats, bran, whole grains, and any other food that is high in fiber. The fiber is what slows down the rate of digestion, and this is what you want in order to avoid big blood sugar surges. Complex carbohydrates, fats, and proteins should be the bulk of your diet in order to minimize the chances of developing this and most other lifestyle-related diseases.

Eating for Health, Eating to Win

The meal plans that I have designed lead you in the right direction for improving your health, minimizing the chances of developing chronic diseases, and looking and feeling better. Once you are on the path toward achieving your health and fitness goals, you will eventually need a customized meal plan and workout in order to bring your health and body to the next level. Meals and workouts that are custom-engineered for you, depending on your body type, fitness goals, tastes and interests, and lifestyle will facilitate the process of reaching your fitness goals. People have different body types, goals, and lifestyles. How could one meal plan and exercise program work for everyone? It isn't possible. This is why I am a strong believer of planning and constructing specific meal plans and exercise programs for each individual and frequently adjusting them along the way. As your body changes throughout the process, your workouts and meal plans should change as well.

32: Sleep

Sleep is a vital part of our lives. Having an adequate amount of sleep on a daily basis is vitally important, especially for kids and teenagers.Sufficient sleep allows your body to function properly. When your body gets proper rest, all its hormones work efficiently and properly. However, when your body doesn't get enough sleep, it suffers internally. Hormone levels get out of balance. Testosterone goes down, for instance, which leads to feeling depressed, having less strength and physical energy, and feeling less confident. Decreasing levels of testosterone are an athlete's worst nightmare. Without the aggression, strength, and confidence testosterone provides, your ability to win goes way down. Testosterone is among the key hormones you need to effectively exercise, win, and feel great mentally.

Another negative effect of insufficient sleep is that your body releases a stress hormone called cortisol. This is one of your "fight or flight" hormones. When cortisol is released, your body's metabolism slows down, your testosterone level decreases, and your body begins to store fat, consuming its own muscle tissue for energy instead. I am sure you can see how none of this is good!

Not sleeping enough also causes a decrease in cognitive function. Without sufficient sleep your brain simply isn't as sharp, your memory isn't as good, and your patience is decreased. Aside from these side effects, your mood is much more depressed. state. In other words, the last thing that you would want to do is not sleep enough! In my personal experience, I know what happens to my body whenever I don't sleep enough. Physically, I am much more tired and when I do exercise, my strength is decreased. When I lift weights, I don't really feel the pump, which is the lactic acid buildup that you feel in the muscle that you are exercising after a few sets. That pump or burn is the feeling we always aim for, because it means you're having a good workout. Mentally, whenever I don't sleep enough I feel sluggish, my memory is poor, my decisions are executed more slowly, and my patience is decreased. I am much more irritable and depressed, and overall I feel as though I am having a really bad day. This is not a good feeling at all!

Please make every effort to get enough sleep. It will really increase your success rate in achieving your physical and mental goals and increase your overall performance and quality of life. Everyone varies in how much sleep is needed, but most people need between seven and eight hours a night to feel at their best.

33: Putting It All Together

The final stage of achieving your fitness goals comes down to knowing when to eat and when to exercise. This all depends on exactly what you are looking to achieve with your body, whether it is that you want to gain or lose weight or compete in sports (and if so, which sport). Knowing what to eat is just as important as knowing when to eat, and the same applies to exercising: knowing which exercises to do and when to do them. The careful timing of meals and exercise can really be precise. There are certain times of the day when you are more hungry than others, and there are certain times of the day when you also have more energy; as well as certain times of the day when you feel more tired. The process of really figuring out your body and how it works can only be achieved with time. While continuing to eat right and exercise you will slowly but surely figure your body out, learning the best times to exercise and eat either higher or lower calorie meals. We all need to start somewhere. Begin by following the program that I lay out below. As you get to know your response, make small adjustments that will further improve your results. The main part of this is starting; the sooner the better. You will need to make adjustments to facilitate your process of getting into shape. It doesn't happen overnight. So why not make this transition as simple and enjoyable as possible, because it can be done!

Daily Menu for the Overweight Child

This menu plan assumes your child is exercising every day by playing outside, riding a bike, playing sports, or working out in some other way. Make sure your child drinks two to three quarts of water or sugar-free beverages every day.

Breakfast	1/2 cup scrambled egg whites
	1 fruit
Snack	1 cup nonfat Greek yogurt with blueberries
Lunch	grilled turkey breast sandwich on rye bread
Snack	1 apple or other fruit
Dinner:	4 oz. grilled chicken breast
	green salad
	sugar-free jello

Daily Menu for the Underweight Child

This menu plan assumes your child is exercising every day by playing outside, riding a bike, playing sports, or working out in some other way. Make sure your child drinks two to three quarts of water or sugar-free beverages every day.

Breakfast	1/2 cup egg whites scrambled with 1 whole omega-3 egg
	1/2 cup of oatmeal
	1 glass all-natural orange juice
Snack	peanut butter and jelly sandwich on whole-wheat bread
Lunch	light tuna in water with low-calorie mayonnaise mixed with chopped vegetables
Snack	2 tablespoons almond butter
Dinner	5 oz. London broil
	1 sweet potato with sour cream
	sugar-free rice pudding
Snack	1/2 cup egg whites scrambled with 1 whole omega-3 egg and low-fat cheese

Daily Menu for the Overweight Vegetarian Child

This menu plan assumes your child is exercising every day by playing outside, riding a bike, playing sports, or working out in some way. Make sure your child drinks two to three quarts of water or sugar-free beverages every day.

Breakfast	1 scoop whey protein isolate blended with fruit and 1/2 cup oats
Snack	carrot and celery sticks with nonfat dip
Lunch	light tuna mixed with mustard and chopped vegetables
Snack	1 fruit
Dinner:	5 oz. grilled fish
	1 cup whole-grain pasta with grated low-fat cheese and olive oil
	green salad
	1 cup sugar-free fruit cocktail

Daily Menu for the Underweight Vegetarian Child

This menu plan assumes your child is exercising every day by playing outside, riding a bike, playing sports, or working out in some way. Make sure your child drinks two to three quarts of water or sugar-free beverages every day.

Breakfast	2 high-fiber waffles with peanut butter and fruit spread
	1/2 cup egg whites scrambled with low-fat cheese
	1 glass all-natural juice
Snack	1/2 cup walnuts
Lunch	1 can salmon with low-calorie mayonnaise on whole-grain bread
Snack	peanut butter and jelly sandwich on high-fiber English muffin
Dinner	5 oz. grilled fish
	1 cup wild rice with olive oil

	steamed vegetables with melted low-fat sharp cheese
	avocado salad
	sugar-free pudding
Snack	low-fat grilled cheese sandwich on whole-grain bread

Daily Menu for the Overweight Vegan Child

This menu plan assumes your child is exercising every day by playing outside, riding a bike, playing sports, or working out in some way. Make sure your child drinks two to three quarts of water or sugar-free beverages every day.

Breakfast	1 scoop soy protein isolate blended with fruit and 1/2 cup old-fashioned oats
Snack	1 fruit
Lunch	brown rice with steamed lentils, fresh tomato sauce, chopped celery
Snack	1 apple
Dinner	extra-firm tofu cooked with vegetables and red beans
	tomato and onion salad with vinegar and olive oil
	fresh fruit cup

Daily Menu for the Underweight Vegan Child

This menu plan assumes your child is exercising every day by playing outside, riding a bike, playing sports, or working out in some way. Make sure your child drinks two to three quarts of water or sugar-free beverages every day.

| Breakfast | 1/2 cup old-fashioned oats with almonds and strawberries mixed with 1 scoop of soy protein isolate |

Snack	mixed nuts and 1 fruit
Lunch	wild rice mixed with black beans and tomato sauce with 1 slice high-fiber bread
Snack	peanut butter and jelly sandwich on whole-grain bread
Dinner:	tofu with baked vegetables
	sweet potato
	fruit cup
Snack	1 scoop soy protein isolate and 1 tablespoon of peanut butter

Daily Menu for the Overweight Teenager

This menu plan assumes your teen is exercising every day by riding a bike, running, playing sports, or working out in some way. Make sure your teen drinks two to three quarts of water or sugar-free beverages every day.

Breakfast	protein shake with 1 scoop whey protein isolate, 1/2 cup oat bran, 1 small fruit, ice, and water all blended together
Snack	1 glass nonfat milk
Lunch	egg white omelet with spinach and mushrooms (2/3 cup egg whites)
Snack	1 fruit
Dinner	chicken parmigiana with nonfat cheese and salt-free tomato sauce
	Greek salad
	steamed vegetables with nonfat cheese
	fresh fruit cup with nonfat whipped cream

Daily Menu for the Underweight Teenager

This menu plan assumes your teen is exercising every day by riding a bike, running, playing sports, or working out in some way. Make sure your teen drinks two to three quarts of water or sugar-free beverages every day.

Breakfast	2 pancakes made with old-fashioned oats, honey, skim milk, served with peanut butter and nonfat whipped cream
	1/2 cup scrambled egg whites
Snack	avocado salad with lettuce, onions, tomato, olive oil, and vinegar
Lunch	low-fat grilled cheese sandwich on whole-wheat bread
	small Greek salad
Snack	1 cup nonfat Greek yogurt with almonds and blueberries
Dinner	grilled London broil with onion and mushrooms
	1 cup whole-grain pasta with low-fat cheese and olive oil
	steamed vegetables or garden salad
	sugar-free, nonfat frozen yogurt
Snack	1 cup nonfat Greek yogurt

Daily Menu for the Vegetarian Overweight Teenager

This menu plan assumes your teen is exercising every day by riding a bike, running, playing sports, or working out in some way. Make sure your teen drinks two to three quarts of water or sugar-free beverages every day.

Breakfast	cheese blintz with nonfat cheese
	1/2 cup scrambled egg whites with mixed vegetables

Snack	1 fruit
Lunch	broiled salmon with lemon and olive oil
	steamed mixed vegetables with grated
	nonfat cheese
Snack	1 cup low-fat cottage cheese with pineapple
Dinner	broiled fish with onions and olive oil
	steamed vegetables with olive oil and
	black pepper
	garden salad with olive oil, vinegar
	and black pepper
	nonfat, sugar-free rice pudding

Daily Menu for the Vegetarian Underweight Teenager

This menu plan assumes your teen is exercising every day by riding a bike, running, playing sports, or working out in some way. Make sure your teen drinks two to three quarts of water or sugar-free beverages every day.

Breakfast	2 high-fiber waffles with peanut butter and
	nonfat whipped cream
	1/2 cup egg whites scrambled with 1 whole
	omega-3 egg and vegetables
	1 glass all-natural fresh juice
Snack	1 low-fat, high-fiber protein bar
Lunch	light tuna in water mixed with onion and
	light mayonnaise in a whole-grain pita
	bread with 1 slice low-fat cheese
Snack	1 apple with 2 tablespoons all-natural
	peanut butter
Dinner	steamed lobster with lemon and butter
	or grilled shrimp with garlic and olive oil
	baked potato with olive oil and garlic
	sautéed vegetables with onion
	and mushrooms

	sugar- and fat-free ice cream
Snack	egg whites scrambled with1 whole omega-3 egg, vegetables, low-fat cheese

Daily Menu for the Overweight Vegan Teenager

This menu plan assumes your teen is exercising every day by riding a bike, running, playing sports, or working out in some way. Make sure your teen drinks two to three quarts of water or sugar-free beverages every day.

Breakfast	protein shake made with 1 scoop soy protein isolate, 1/3 cup oat bran, 1 small banana, ice, and water
Snack	fresh fruit cup
Lunch	salad with onion, tomato, garbanzo beans, olive oil, vinegar with 1 high-fiber pita bread
Snack	1 glass nonfat soy milk
Dinner	sautéed vegetables with onion, tofu, tomato, green pepper and mushroom lentil soup garden salad with flaxseeds 1 cup grapes

Daily Menu for the Underweight Vegan Teenager

This menu plan assumes your teen is exercising every day by riding a bike, running, playing sports, or working out in some way. Make sure your teen drinks two to three quarts of water or sugar-free beverages every day.

Breakfast	1 high-fiber, low-carb English muffin with almond butter and sugar-free, high-fiber fruit preserves 1 banana 1 glass nonfat rice milk

Snack	3 rice cakes with peanut butter
Lunch:	1 cup whole-grain pasta mixed with black beans and lentils, olive oil
	sautéed green beans with olive oil, black pepper, garlic
Snack	1 glass low-fat soy milk
	1 cup strawberries
Dinner	mashed sweet potato mixed with nonfat soy milk and 1 scoop soy protein isolate
	garden salad with walnuts and olive oil
	fresh fruit cup
Snack	1 glass nonfat rice milk mixed with 1 scoop soy protein isolate

It is important to remember that improving your body is a process that won't happen overnight. It is extremely important for you to follow one of the meal plans for an extended period of time so you will see results. This is a lifestyle, not just a diet or an exercise routine. The results will only come through consistent hard work and discipline every day. This is why I like to compare this to a marathon, rather than a 100-meter sprint. There is no question that you will see the results of your hard work. When they come, you will realize that the work involved was well worth it and has definitely paid off. Being in shape is a feeling that no amount of money could ever buy. Feeling great, looking great, and winning in sports are awesome natural highs that are achieved only from following a constant and steady meal and workout plan just like the few examples that I have given you.

My knowledge comes not only from constant research but through experience, too. I want you to know that following these meal plans is just a start. Once you get the idea, you can make changes in the meals to accommodate your tastes and the changes in your body. I strongly believe that each person should have their daily workout and meal itineraries custom-made for them depending on their taste in food, choices of exercises, fitness goals, and lifestyles. Specifically designing your exercise and meal plan will further your chances of not only adhering to the plan for a longer period of time, but also enjoying the process.

Having fun is really what it's all about! We must enjoy whatever we do in order to do it well. It's all about passion, quality of life, and most of all, achieving results. You must really want to make the commitment to improving your body and athletic performance for this to work. Please, never wait for tomorrow. Never use excuses to stop you from achieving your dreams. Never think that any dream is impossible to achieve. Achieving your dream takes hard work, commitment, perseverance, desire, dedication, and determination. Once you combine these, your dreams now become reality. One of the greatest feelings of all is taking a dream, an idea, a vision, and turning it into a reality! Dreams don't have expiration dates! Start working on them now so that you will have that body you dream of, or you will be that champion athlete. These goals are within your reach and for the taking. Setbacks will come along the way, but never let these small obstacles stop you. Our character is best tested only when we are faced with adversity. Proceed forward no matter what! When you believe, you shall achieve. Always remember that life is short and youth is even shorter. Never wait: execute your plan now. The sooner your dreams turn to reality, the happier you will be. Nothing will give you a greater smile than success!